ILLUSTRATIONS OF SPECIAL EFFECTIVE ACUPOINTS

for common diseases

This book is one of four in the series;
Quick Reference Handbooks of Chinese Medicine

Editor

Guo Changqing & Liu Naigang

Published by

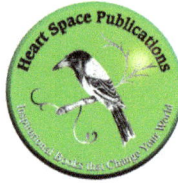

Heart Space Publications
PO Box 1085
Daylesford
Victoria
3460
Australia
Tel +61 450260348
www.heartspacebooks.com
pat@heartspacebooks.com

Published in 2021 at Melbourne

Medical information disclaimer – Although these practices have proven themselves over eons, it is always a good idea to consult with your registered doctor or registered health practitioner for any medical concerns. Always consider your medical officers advice first. As the publisher of this manual, we make no warranties or claims, or make any representations or warranties, express or implied as to the validity of these practices.

ISBN 978-0-6489215-9-2

CONTENTS

Abstract

The book is compiled and edited by senior specialists and professors of the School of Acupuncture, Moxibustion, and Massage of Beijing University of Chinese Medicine. It selects acupuncture points that have special effects on some diseases, and gives standard location and indications of the points, especially the specific acupuncture points in both Chinese and English. With clear illustrations as assistance, the book helps readers precisely locate the points. The book is applicable to both teachers and students of TCM colleges and universities, clinical practitioners, and amateurs.

Testimonial

Specific acupuncture points are broadly used in acupuncture clinics, and are the most effective acupoints when it comes to treating common conditions. This book includes all of the specific acupoints, including Five-shu points, Yuan-source points, Luo-connecting points, Back shu points, Front mu points, Eight confluence points, Eight influential points, Xi-cleft points, and Lower he-sea points. This book contains not only accurate and concise descriptions of the locations and indications of these points, but is also accompanied by clear illustrations that allow the reader to easily locate acupoints. This is a very good handbook for clinical acupuncturists, Chinese medical school students and Chinese medicine amateurs to guide their clinical practices and studies.

Yueping Li, PhD of Chinese medicine
Australian registered Chinese Medical doctor and Acupuncturist

Preface

Acupuncture therapy takes acupuncture points as the foundation. All its therapeutic effects are obtained by the stimulation of the points. Therefore, the study of acupuncture points plays an important role in the study of acupuncture. Among all the acupuncture points, specific acupuncture points are of utmost importance. Specific acupuncture points refer to points of the fourteen meridians and of the therapeutic effects and titles, including five-shu points, yuan-source points, luo-connecting points, xi-cleft points, back-shu point, front-mu point, lower he-sea points of the six fu organs, eight influential points, and confluence points of the eight extraordinary vessels.

Specific acupuncture points have far more effective curative effects than the others. Therefore, to be familiar with and master the knowledge of specific acupuncture points is the necessary basis for the study and application of acupuncture therapy, as well as the essential condition for a satisfactory clinical curative effect.

The book is mainly for the introduction of standard locations and indications of all the specific acupuncture points. It narrates with illustrations as assistance for the readers' convenience on the locating and clinical application of specific acupuncture points. We hope that the publication of the book will help with the clinical use of specific acupuncture points.

Editor
April, 2010

CHAPTER 1

Methods of Locating Special Acupuncture Points

Section 1
Finger-length Measurement

Finger measurement is a method of standard measurement, for the location of the acupuncture point, since the fingers are in proportion with the other parts of the body – that the length and width of the patient's fingers are taken.

1. Four Measurement

The width of the four fingers (index, middle, ring and little) placed together, taken at the level of the dorsal crease of the proximal interphalangeal joint of the middle finger measures 3 cun. Cun is the term for the measurement relative to the patient (see images below). This method is always used to locate the points in the abdomen, back and lower limbs.

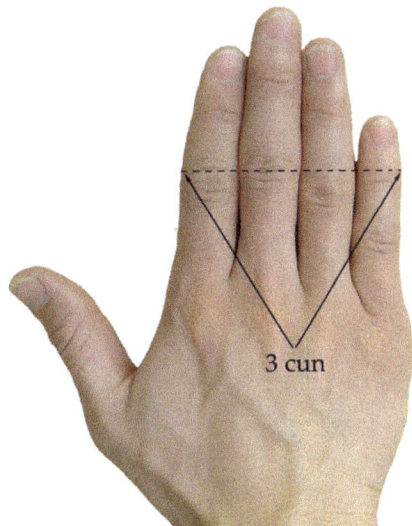

3 cun

2. Thumb Measurement

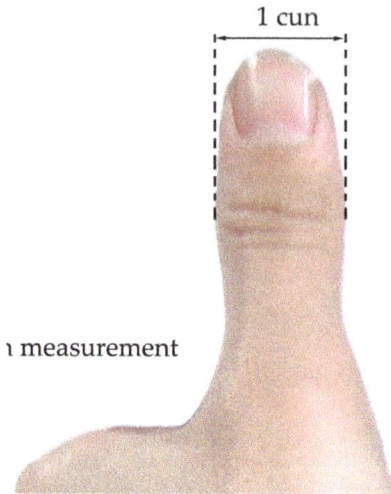

1 cun

Place the thumb straight. The width of the interphalangeal joint of the patient's thumb is 1 cun.

ı measurement

3. Middle Finger Measurement

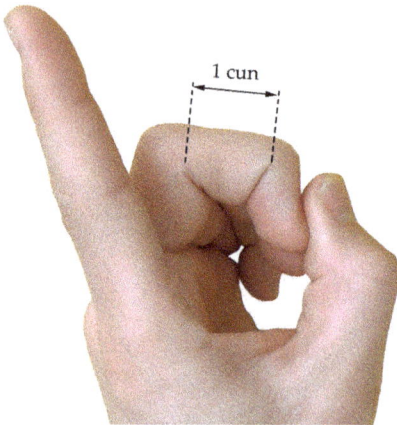

1 cun

When the patient's middle finger is flexed, the index finger is straight, and the end of the middle finger against the belly of the thumb, forming a ring. The width between the two medial ends of the creases of the interphalangeal joints is 1 cun. This method is suitable for limbs and transverse measurement of the dorsal.

Section 2
Bone-Length Measurement

The commonly used modern method of orientation of "bony degree" is based on Ling Shu (superior pivot), and in the long-term medical practice after modification and supplement, see the table below for details.

Standard for Bone-Length Measurement

Body Part	Area between two points on the body	Length in cun
Head	From the midpoint of the anterior hairline to the midpoint of the posterior hairline	12 cun

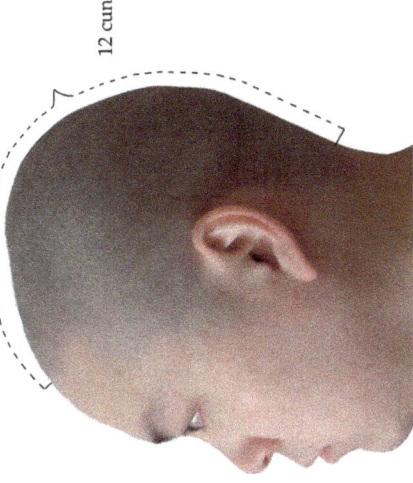

12 cun

Head	Between the corners of the forehead ST 8.	9 cun
Head	Between the two mastoid processes	9 cun
Chest and Abdomen	From the suprasternal fossa to the sternocostal angle	9 cun
	From the sternocostal angle to the center of the umbilicus	8 cun
	From the center of the umbilicus to the upper of symphysis pubis	5 cun
	Between the two nipples	8 cun

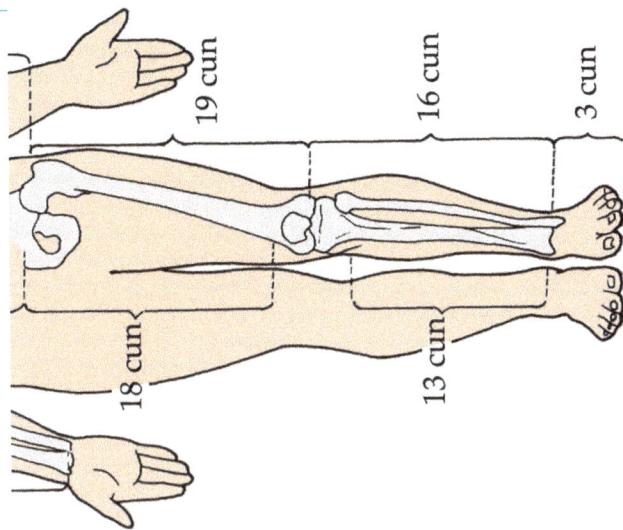

Lateral side of the trunk	From the tip of the axillary fossa to the tip of the 11th rib.	12 cun
	From the tip of the 11th rib to the prominence of the great trochanter	9 cun
Upper Limbs	From the end of the axillary fold to the transverse cubital crease	9 cun
	From the transverse cubital crease to the transverse wrist crease	12 cun
Lower Limbs	From the level of the border of symphysis pubis to the medial epicondyle of the femur	18 cun
	From the lower border of the medial condyle of tibia to the tip of medial malleolus	13 cun
	From the prominence of the great trochanter to the middle of patella	19 cun
	From the center of patella to the tip of lateral malleolus	16 cun
	From the tip of lateral malleolus to the sole.	3 cun

Illustrations of Special Effective Acupoints • 5

CHAPTER 2

Five-shu Points

Section I
Points of Lung Meridian of Hand Taiyin: LU

LU-11 Shàoshāng — Jing-well point of LU

[Action]	Relieves the surface and clears heat, relieves sore-throat and revives consciousness.
[Position]	On the radial side of the thumb, 0.1 cun lateral to the corner of the nail.
[Acupuncture and Moxibustion]	**Acupuncture:** Insert the needle subcutaneously 0.1~0.2 cun deep: Or prick with three-edged needle and press tightly to bleed. **Moxibustion:** Apply 1~3 moxa cones or place a moxa stick above the point for 5-10 minutes.
[Indications]	Cough, asthma, sore throat, epistaxis and chest distention. Coma, loss of consciousness, epilepsy and infantile convulsion, vomiting. Spasmodic pain of the thumb and the wrist, fever.

LU-10 Yújì — Ying-spring point of LU

[Action]	Relieves the surface and clears heat, disperses lung Qi and relieves sore-throat.
[Position]	In the depression proximal to the metacarpo-phalangeal joint, on the radial side of the midpoint of the metacarpal bone, at the junction of the red and white skin.
[Acupuncture and Moxibustion]	**Acupuncture:** Insert the needle perpendicularly 0.3~0.5 cun deep. Or prick with a three-edged needle to bleed. **Moxibustion:** Apply 3-5 moxa cones or place a moxa stick above the point for 3-5 minutes.
[Indications]	Swelling and pain in the throat.

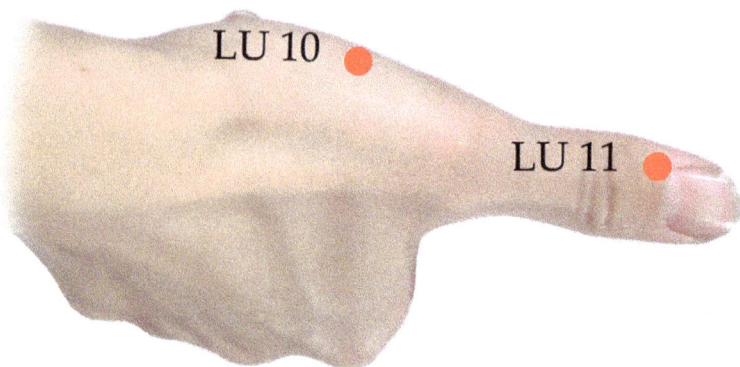

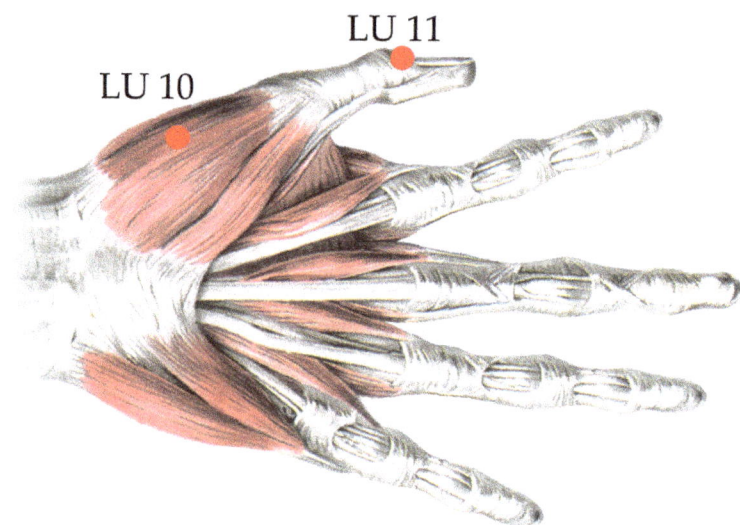

LU-9 Tàiyuān — Shu-stream point of LU: Influential point of the vessels: Yuan-source of LU

[Action]	Alleviates cough and transforms phlegm, regulates and harmonizes the vessels, tonifies Qi and invigorates the spleen.
[Position]	On the radial end of the wrist crease, in depression ulnar to the m. abductor pollicis longus, between the styloid process of radius and scaphoid bone
[Acupuncture and Moxibustion]	**Acupuncture:** Insert the needle perpendicularly 0.2~0.3 cun deep. Avoid puncturing the radial artery. **Moxibustion:** Apply 1-3 moxa cones or place a moxa stick above the point for 5-10 minutes.
[Indications]	Cough, asthma, chest congestion, palpitations and pulseless disease.

LU-8 Jīngqú — Jing-river point of LU

[Action]	Disperses lung Qi and alleviates wheezing, regulates Qi in the chest.
[Position]	On the radial side of the palmar surface of the forearm, 1 cun proximal to the transverse crease of the wrist, in the depression between the styloid process of the radius and the radial artery.
[Acupuncture and Moxibustion]	**Acupuncture:** Insert the needle perpendicularly 0.1~0.3 cun deep. Avoid puncturing the radial artery. **Moxibustion:** Apply 3~5 moxa cones or place a moxa stick above the point for 5~10 minutes.
[Indications]	Cough, asthma, chest congestion, pain of the chest and back, pharyngitis, heat in centre of the palm and pulseless disease.

LU-5 Chǐzé — He-sea point of LU

[Action]	Descends rebellious Qi and alleviates cough, nourishes yin and moisturizes lung
[Position]	On the radial side of the tendon of m. biceps brachii at the level of the transverse cubital crease.
[Acupuncture and Moxibustion]	**Acupuncture:** Insert the needle perpendicularly 0.5~1.0 cun deep. Prick with a three-edged needle to bleed. **Moxibustion:** apply 5-7 moxa cones or needle-warming moxibustion or place a moxa stick above the point for 5-10 minutes.
[Indications]	Cough, asthma, hemoptysis, sore throat, chest distention, infantile convulsion, vomiting and diarrhea, spasmodic pain of the elbow and arm.

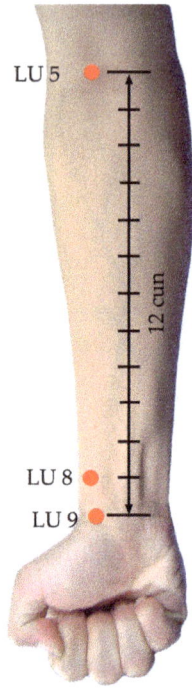

LU 5

12 cun

LU 8
LU 9

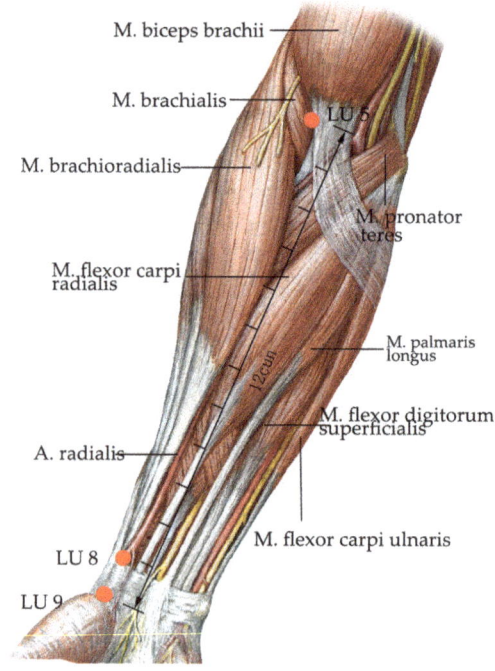

M. biceps brachii

M. brachialis

LU 5

M. brachioradialis

M. pronator teres

M. flexor carpi radialis

M. palmaris longus

M. flexor digitorum superficialis

A. radialis

M. flexor carpi ulnaris

12 cun

LU 8
LU 9

Section II
Points of Intestine Meridian of Hand Yangming: LI

LI-1 Shāngyáng — Jing-well point of LI

[Action]	Relieves the surface and clears heat and revives consciousness.
[Position]	On the radial side of the index finger, 0.1 cun medial to the corner of the nail.
[Acupuncture and Moxibustion]	**Acupuncture:** Insert the needle perpendicularly 0.1~0.2 cun deep: Or prick with a three-edged needle to bleed. **Moxibustion:** Apply 1-3 moxa cones or place a moxa stick above the point for 5-10 minutes.
[Indications]	Pharyngitis, fainting, stroke with loss consciousness and febrile diseases with anhidrosis.

LI-2 Erjiān — Ying-spring point of LI

[Action]	Relieves the surface and clears heat and relieves sore-throat.
[Position]	On the radial side of the index finger, in the depression distal to the metacarpalphalangeal joint, at the junction of the red and white skin when the hand is in a loose fist.
[Acupuncture and Moxibustion]	**Acupuncture:** Insert the needle perpendicularly 0.2~0.4 cun deep **Moxibustion:** Apply3-5 moxa cones or place a moxa stick above the point for 5-10 minutes.
[Indications]	Swelling and pain in the throat, toothache and prosopalgia.

LI-3 Sānjiān — Shu-stream point of LI

[Action]	Clears heat, relieves pain and benefits the throat.
[Position]	On the radial side of the index finger, in the depression proximal to the head of the second metacarpal bone when the hand is in a loose fist.
[Acupuncture and Moxibustion]	**Acupuncture:** Insert the needle perpendicularly 0.3~0.5 cun deep **Moxibustion:** Apply 3-5 moxa cones or place a moxa stick above the point for 5-10 minutes.
[Indications]	Swelling and pain in the throat, chest distention and fever

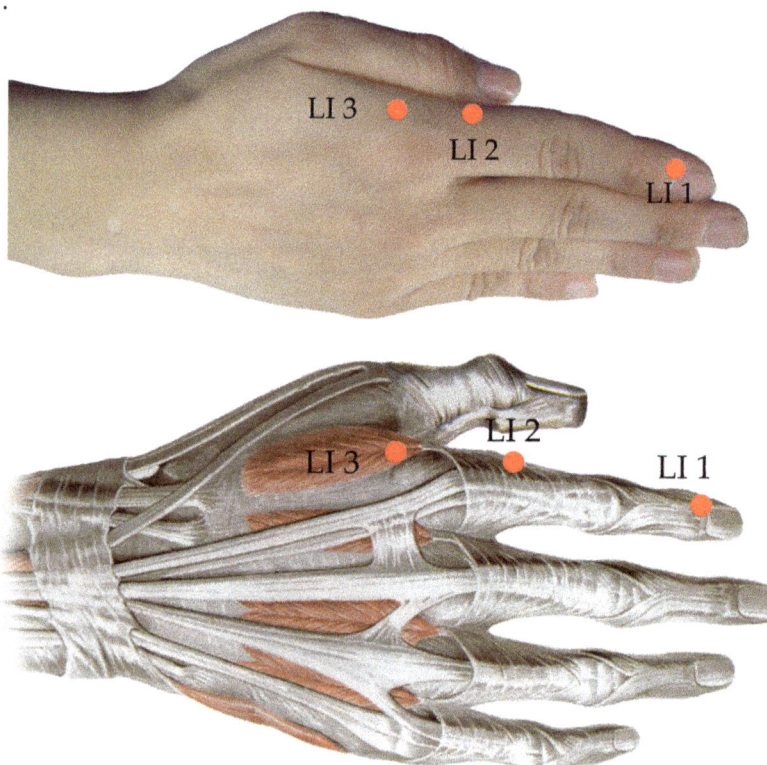

LI-5 Yángxī — Jing-river point of LI

[Action]	Expels wind and clears heat, benefits the wrist joint.
[Position]	On the dorsal side of the wrist, in the depression between the tendons of m. extensor pollicis longus and m. extensor pollicis brevis when the thumb is pointing upward.
[Acupuncture and Moxibustion]	**Acupuncture:** Insert the needle perpendicularly 0.5~0.8 cun deep. **Moxibustion:** Apply3-5 moxa cones or place a moxa stick above the point for 10-20 minutes.
[Indications]	Sore throat, redness, swelling and pain of the eye, fever and upset.

LI-11 Qûchí — He-sea point of LI

[Action]	Clears heat and expels wind, regulates Qi and blood and activates collaterals to relieve pain.
[Position]	In the depression of the radial side of the transverse cubital crease when elbow flexed, midway between LU5 (Chǐzé) and the lateral epicondyle of the humerus.
[Acupuncture and Moxibustion]	**Acupuncture:** Insert the needle perpendicularly 1.0~2.5 cun deep **Moxibustion:** Apply 5-7 moxa cones or place a moxa stick above the point for 5-20 minutes.
[Indications]	Swelling and pain of throat, cough, asthma, fever, vomiting and diarrhea, abdominal pain, dysentery, intestinal carbuncle, constipation, toothache, pain and redness of the eyes, itrismus epilepsy, measles, sores, scabies, exanthemata, erysipelas, redness and swelling of the arm redness, paralysis of the upper limb, pain and paralysis of the elbow and shoulder and high blood pressure.

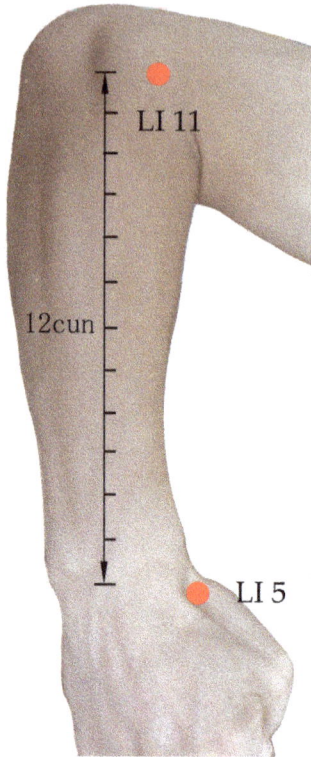
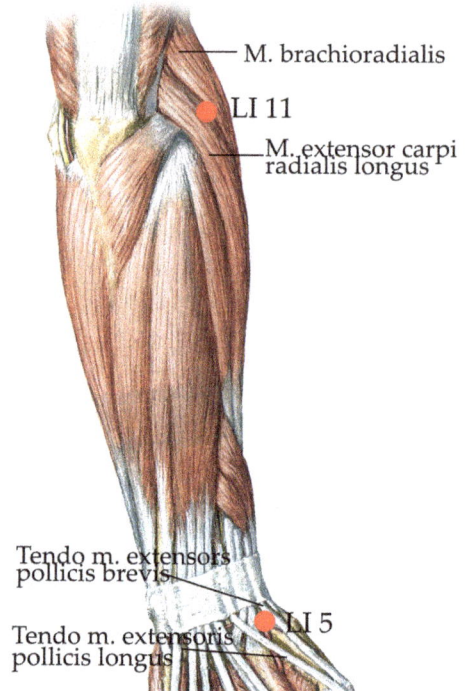

LI 11

12cun

LI 5

M. brachioradialis

LI 11

M. extensor carpi radialis longus

Tendo m. extensors pollicis brevis

Tendo m. extensoris pollicis longus

LI 5

Section III
Points of Stomach Meridian of Foot Yangming: ST

ST-45 Lìduì — Jing-well point of ST

[Action]	Clears heat of the stomach channel, calms the spirit and restores consciousness, dredges the channel and actives the collaterals.
[Position]	On the lateral side of the second toe, 0.1 cun lateral to the corner of the nail.
[Acupuncture and Moxibustion]	**Acupuncture:** Insert the needle subcutaneously 0.1~0.2 cun deep: Or prick with three-edged needle to bleed. **Moxibustion:** Apply 1-3 moxa cones or place a moxa stick above the point for 5~10 minutes.
[Indications]	Toothache, profuse dreaming, febrile diseases and mental diseases.

ST-44 Nèitíng — Ying-spring point of ST

[Action]	Clears fire of the stomach channel, regulates Qi and alleviates pain.
[Position]	On the dorsum of foot, in distal to the second metatarsophalangeal joint, in the web between the second and third toes.
[Acupuncture and Moxibustion]	**Acupuncture:** Insert the needle perpendicularly or obliquely 0.3~0.5 cun deep **Moxibustion:** Apply 3-5 moxa cones or place a moxa stick above the point for 5~10 minutes.
[Indications]	Disorders of the stomach and intestines: Abdominal pain and distention, diarrhea and dysentery. Toothache, head and face pain, deviated mouth, pharyngitis, epistaxis, irritability, insomnia with many dreams, psychosis, swelling and pain in the dorsum of the foot and metatarsophalangeal joints.

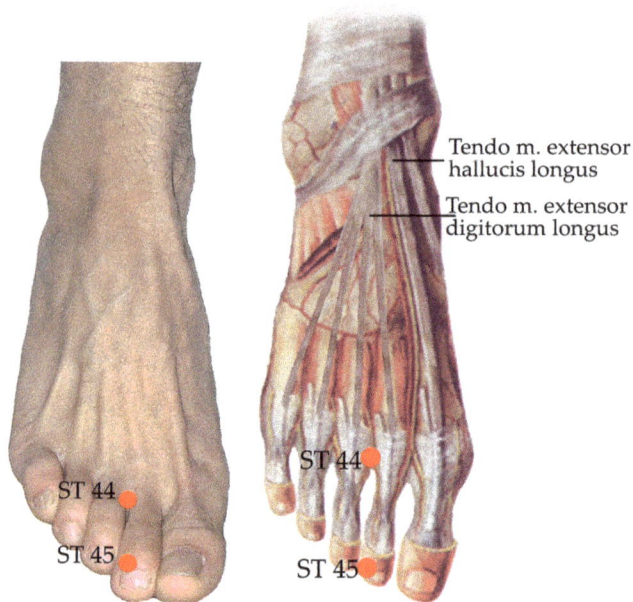

Tendo m. extensor
hallucis longus

Tendo m. extensor
digitorum longus

ST 44

ST 45

ST 44

ST 45

ST-43 Xiàngǔ — Shu-stream point of ST

[Action]	Relieving the exterior pathogens by cooling, harmonizes the stomach and dispels edema and regulates Qi and alleviates pain.
[Position]	On the dorsum of foot, proximal to the second and third metatarsophalangeal joint, in depression distal to the junction of the second and third metatarsal bones.
[Acupuncture and Moxibustion]	**Acupuncture:** Insert the needle perpendicularly 0.2~0.3 cun deep. **Moxibustion:** Apply 3-5 moxa cones or place a moxa stick above the point for 5~10 minutes.
[Indications]	Swollen face, borborygmus and abdominal pain and pain in the dorsum of the foot

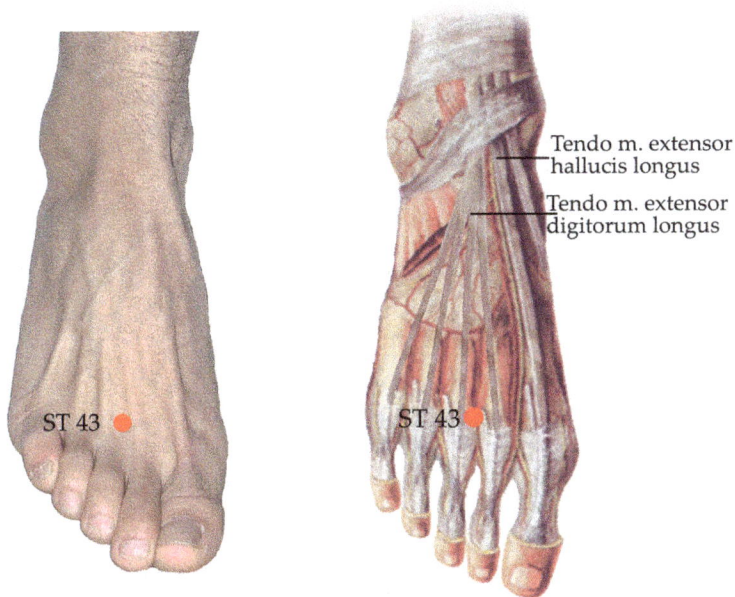

Tendo m. extensor
hallucis longus

Tendo m. extensor
digitorum longus

ST 43

ST 43

ST-41 Jiěxī — Jing-river point of ST

[Action]	Harmonizes the stomach and transforms phlegm, dredges and activates the channel and calms the spirit.
[Position]	In the horizontal stria of the dorsum of foot, between the extensor pollicis longus muscle tendon and the extensor digitorum longus.
[Acupuncture and Moxibustion]	**Acupuncture:** Insert the needle perpendicularly 0.2~0.3 cun deep. **Moxibustion:** Apply 3-5 moxa cones or place a moxa stick above the point for 5~10 minutes.
[Indications]	Headache, abdominal pain, constipation and swelling and pain in the ankle.

ST-36 Zúsānlǐ He-sea point of ST

[Action]	Invigorates the spleen and harmonizes the stomach, prevents disease and benefits macrobiosis, dredges the channel and actives the collaterals, rises and falls Qi.
[Position]	On the anterior aspect of the lower leg, 3 cun distal to ST 35 (Dúbí), one finger width lateral from the anterior ridge of the tibia.
[Acupuncture and Moxibustion]	**Acupuncture:** Insert the needle perpendicularly 0.5~1.5 cun deep. **Moxibustion:** Apply 5-10 moxa cones or place a moxa stick above the point for 10~20 minutes. Pustulating moxibustion and natural moxibustion can be used to promote health and well-being.
[Indications]	Disorders of the stomach and intestines: Stomach ache, vomiting, abdominal distention, borborygmus, indigestion, diarrhea, constipation, dysentery. Disorders of the heart: Irritability, palpitation, insomnia, psychosis, epilepsy and stroke. Wheezing with phlegm, carbuncle weakness and hemoptysis, dysuria, enuresis and hernia. Pain of the knee and shin pain, paralysis of the lower limbs, beriberi, edema:vertigo, deafness, diseases of the nose and eyes, irritability, and insomnia.

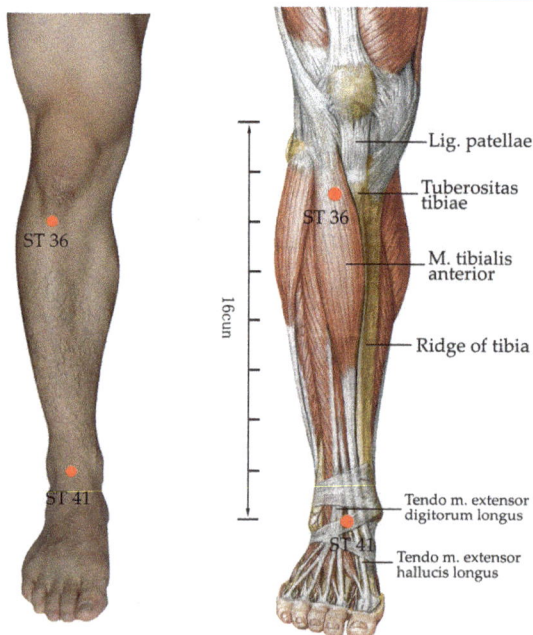

Section IV
Points of Spleen Meridian of Foot Taiyin: SP

SP-1 Yǐnbái — Jing-well point of SP

[Action]	Benefits Qi and stops bleeding, invigorates the spleen, calms the spirit and restores consciousness.
[Position]	On the medial side of the big toe, 0.1 cun lateral to the corner of the nail.
[Acupuncture and Moxibustion]	**Acupuncture:** Insert the needle subcutaneously 0.1~0.2 cun deep: Or prick with the three-edged needle to bleed. **Moxibustion:** Apply1-3 moxa cones or place a moxa stick above the point for 5~10 minutes.
[Indications]	Irregular menstruation, metrorrhagia, abdominal distention, sudden and violent diarrhea, epilepsy, insomnia with many dreams. And the clinical treatment of the blood-proof effect is good.

SP-2 Dàdū — Ying-spring point of SP

[Action]	Invigorates the spleen and harmonizes the middle jiao and clears heat and alleviates pain.
[Position]	On the medial side of foot, in the depression at the junction of the red and white skin anterior and inferior to the proximal metatarsodigital joint of the big toe.
[Acupuncture and Moxibustion]	**Acupuncture:** Insert the needle perpendicularly 0.3~0.5 cun deep. **Moxibustion:** Apply1-3 moxa cones or place a moxa stick above the point for 5~10 minutes.
[Indications]	Abdominal distention and pain and stomachache.

SP-3 Tàibái — Shu-stream point of SP: Yuan-source point of SP

[Action]	Invigorates the spleen and harmonizes the stomach, removes dampness and clears heat.
[Position]	On the medial side of foot, in the depression at the junction of red and white skin, posterior and inferior to the proximal metatarsodigital joint of the big toe.
[Acupuncture and Moxibustion]	**Acupuncture:** Insert the needle perpendicularly 0.3~0.5 cun deep.
	Moxibustion: Apply 1-3 moxa cones or place a moxa stick above the point for 5~10 minutes.
[Indications]	Stomachache, borborygmus, abdominal distention and pain, vomiting and diarrhea.

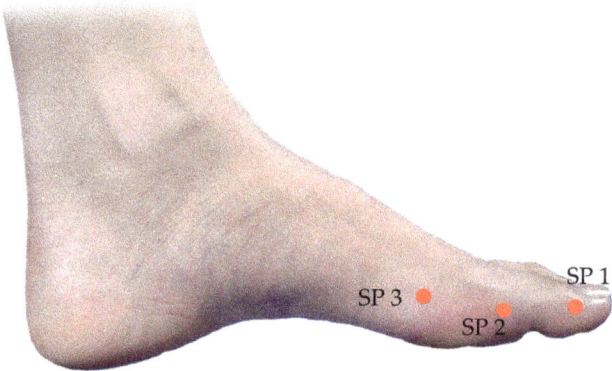

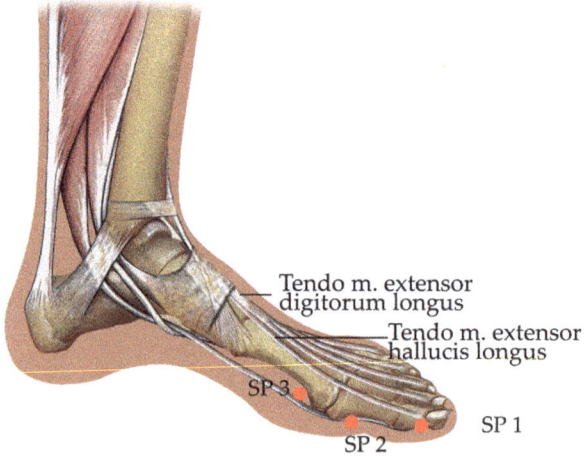

SP 5 Shāngqiū — Jing-river point of SP

[Action]	Invigorates the spleen and resolves dampness: harmonizes the intestines and stomach.
[Position]	In the depression anterior and inferior to the medial malleolus, at the midpoint between the tuberosity of the navicular bone and the tip of the medial malleolus.
[Acupuncture and Moxibustion]	**Acupuncture:** Insert the needle perpendicularly 0.3~0.5 cun deep. **Moxibustion:** Apply 1-3 moxa cones or place a moxa stick above the point for 5~10 minutes.
[Indications]	Paralysis of the lower limbs and ankle pain.

SP-9 Yīnlíngquán — He-sea point of SP

[Action]	Removes dampness and clears heat, invigorates the spleen and regulates Qi, tonifies kidney and regulates menstruation, dredges the channel and actives the collaterals.
[Position]	On the medial part of the lower leg, in the depression of the lower border of the medial condyle of the tibia.
[Acupuncture and Moxibustion]	**Acupuncture:** Insert the needle perpendicularly 1.0~1.5 cun deep **Moxibustion:** Apply 3-5 moxa cones or place a moxa stick above the point for 5~10 minutes.
[Indications]	Abdominal pain and distention, edema, incontinence, enuresis.

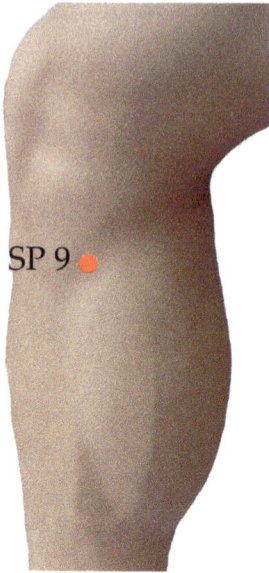

SP 9

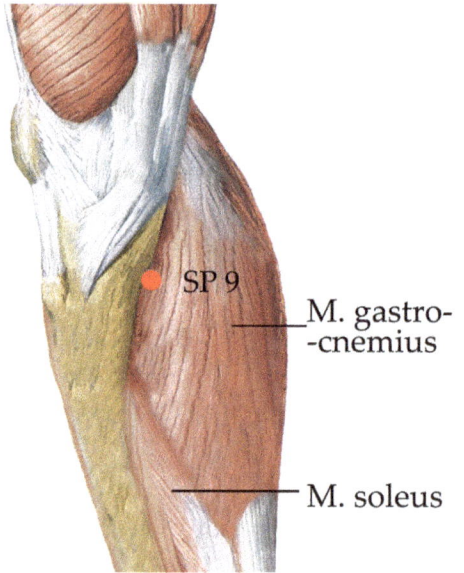

SP 9

M. gastro-
-cnemius

M. soleus

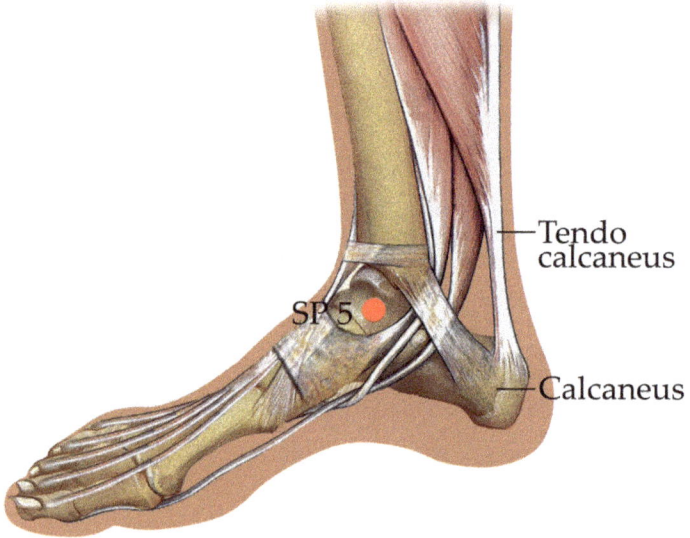

Tendo
calcaneus

SP 5

Calcaneus

Section V
Points of Heart Meridian of Hand Shaoyin: HT

HT-9 Shàochōng — Jing-well point of HT

[Action]	Clears heat and extinguishes wind, calms the spirit and revives consciousness, regulates blood and dredges the channel.
[Position]	On the radial side of the distal aspect of the little finger, 0.1 cun lateral to the radial corner of the nail.
[Acupuncture and Moxibustion]	**Acupuncture:** Insert the needle subcutaneously 0.1~0.2 cun deep: Or prick with the three-edged needle to bleed. **Moxibustion:** Apply 3-5 moxa cones or place a moxa stick above the point for 5~10 minutes.
[Indications]	Psychosis, febrile diseases and epilepsy, stroke and loss of consciousness.

HT-8 Shàofǔ — Ying-spring point of HT

[Action]	Clears heat of the heart, regulates Qi and activates the collateral.
[Position]	In the palm, between the 4th and 5th metacarpal bone. The point is located under the tip of the little finger when the hand makes a loose fist.
[Acupuncture and Moxibustion]	**Acupuncture:** Insert the needle perpendicularly 0.3~0.5 cun deep. **Moxibustion:** Apply 3-5 moxa cones or place a moxa stick above the point for 5~7 minutes.
[Indications]	Heart palpitation, sadness and panic disorder, chest pain, heat in the palm, spasmodic pain of the little finger, pain in the nerve of the arm.

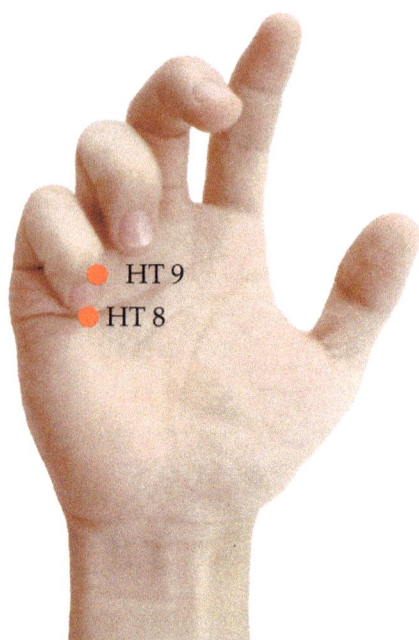

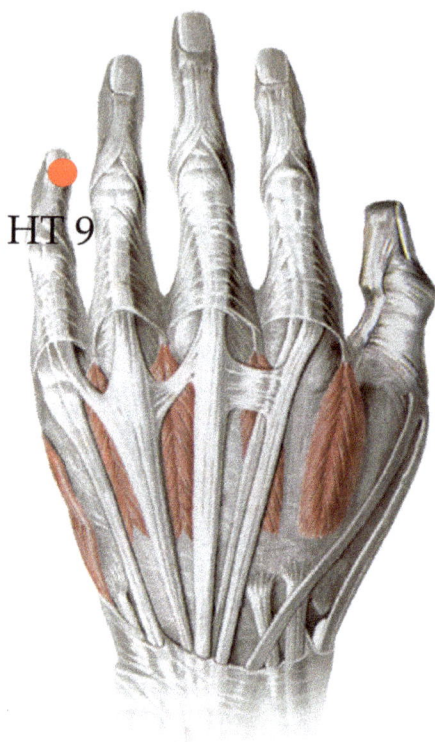

HT 9

HT 9
HT 8

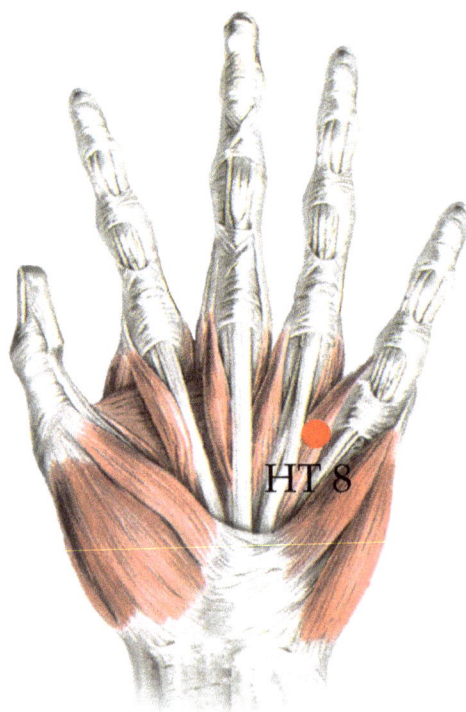

HT 8

HT-7 Shénmén — Shu-stream point of HT: Yuan-source point of HT

[Action]	Tonifies the heart and calms the spirit, dredges the channel and actives the collaterals.
[Position]	On the radial side of the tendon m. flexor carpi ulnaris of the transverse wrist crease.
[Acupuncture and Moxibustion]	**Acupuncture:** Insert the needle perpendicularly 0.3~0.5 cun deep and avoid the ulnar artery and vein. **Moxibustion:** Apply 3-5 moxa cones or place a moxa stick above the point for 5~15minutes.
[Indications]	Irritability, cardiac pain, palpitation, amnesia, insomnia, dementia, psychosis, epilepsy, headache, vertigo, pharyngxerosis, sudden loss of voice, numbness, pain and cold of the arm, asthma, haematemesis and asitia because of the fever.

HT-4 Língdào — Jing-river point of HT

[Action]	Tonifies the heart and calms the spirit, actives the blood and dredges the collaterals.
[Position]	On the medial aspect of the forearm, on the radial side of the tendon m. flexor carpi ulnaris, 1.5 cun proximal to the transverse wrist crease.
[Acupuncture and Moxibustion]	**Acupuncture:** Insert the needle perpendicularly 0.5~0.8 cun deep and avoid the ulnar artery and vein. **Moxibustion:** Apply 1-3 moxa cones or place a moxa stick above the point for 10~20 minutes.
[Indications]	Cardiac pain and numbness of the hands.

HT-3 Shàohǎi He-sea point of HT

[Action]	Regulates Qi and dredges the collaterals, tonifies the heart and calms the spirit.
[Position]	On the mid-point of the line connecting the medial end of the transverse crease of the elbow to the medial epicondyle of the humerus when the elbow is flexed.
[Acupuncture and Moxibustion]	**Acupuncture:** Insert the needle perpendicularly 0.5~1.0 cun deep and stimulate until there is a sore and numbing sensation in the local area or an electric sensation radiating to the forearm. **Moxibustion:** Apply 3-5 moxa cones or place a moxa stick above the point for 5~10 minutes.
[Indications]	Cardiac pain, psychosis, epilepsy, sudden loss of voice, spasmodic pain and numbness of the elbow and arm.

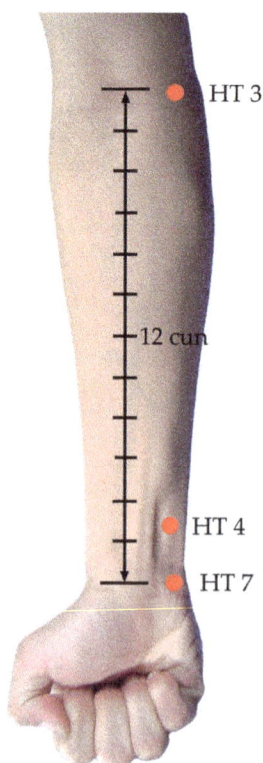

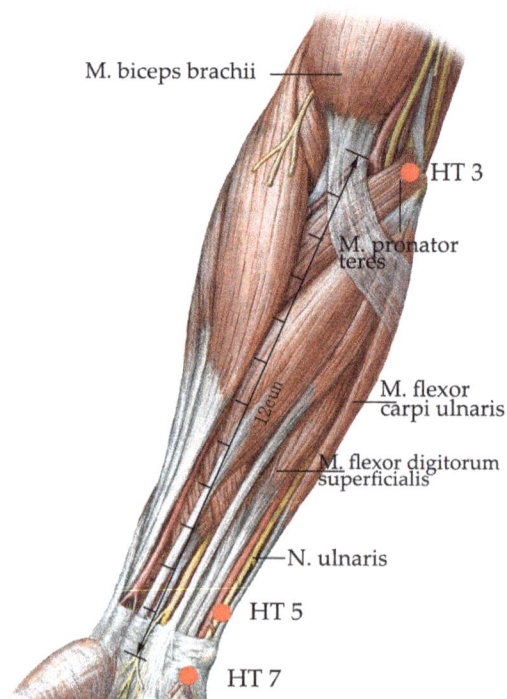

Section VI
Points of Small Intestine Meridian of Hand Taiyang: SI

SI-1 Shàozé — Jing-well point of SI

[Action]	Clears heat and promotes lactation, eliminates stasis and revives consciousness.
[Position]	On the ulnar side of the distal phalanx of the little finger, 0.1 cun lateral to the corner of the nail.
[Acupuncture and Moxibustion]	**Acupuncture:** Insert the needle subcutaneously 0.1~0.2 cun deep: Or prick with the three-edged needle to bleed. **Moxibustion:** Apply 1-3 moxa cones or place a moxa stick above the point for 3~5 minutes.
[Indications]	Stroke and loss of conciseness, superficial visual obstruction and insufficient lactation.

SI-2 Qiángǔ Ying-spring point of SI

[Action]	Relieves superficial excess by cooling, clears the head and brightens the eyes, dredges the channel and actives the collatrals.
[Position]	On the ulnar side of the hand, distal to the fifth metacarpophalangeal joint, at the end of the transverse crease, at the junction of the red and white skin.
[Acupuncture and Moxibustion]	**Acupuncture:** Insert the needle perpendicularly 0.2~0.3 cun deep. **Moxibustion:** Apply 1-3 moxa cones or place a moxa stick above the point for 5~10 minutes.
[Indications]	Pain and rigidity of the head and neck, neck stiffness and arm pain.

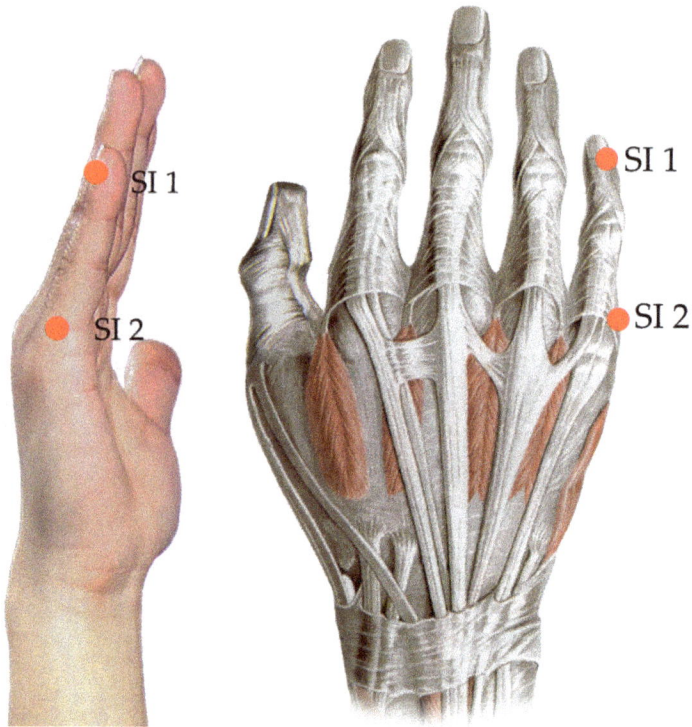

SI 1

SI 2

SI 1

SI 2

SI-3 Hòuxī — Shu-stream point of SI: Confluent points of the Du vessel.

[Action]	Clears the head and brightens the eyes, calms the spirit and treats epilepsy, dredges the channel and actives the collateral.
[Position]	On the ulnar side of the hand, proximal to the fifth metacarpophalangeal joint, at the end of the transverse crease, at the junction of the red and white skin side.
[Acupuncture and Moxibustion]	**Acupuncture:** Insert the needle perpendicularly 0.5~0.8 cun deep. **Moxibustion:** Apply 1-3 moxa cones or place a moxa stick above the point for 5~10 minutes.
[Indications]	Febrile diseases with anhidrosis, jaundice, malaria, painful eyes and lacrimation, superficial visual obstruction, swelling of cheeks, swollen and sore throat, psychosis, epilepsy, hysteria, insomnia, stroke, pain and rigidity of the head and neck, spasmodic pain and numbness of the elbow, arm and little finger, paralysis

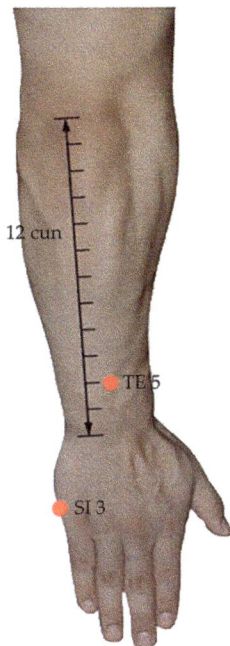

12 cun

TE 5

SI 3

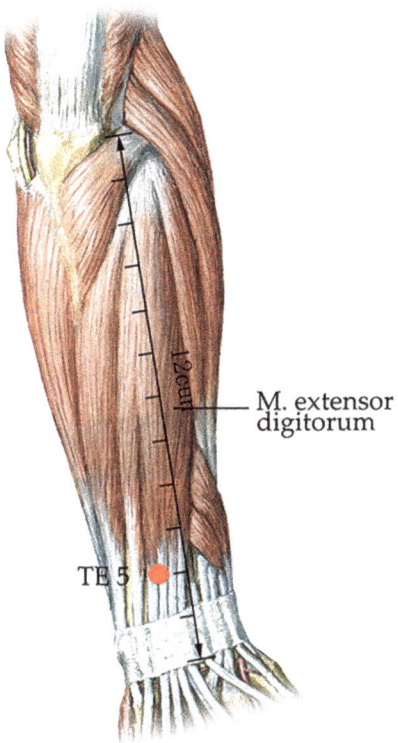

M. extensor digitorum

12cun

TE 5

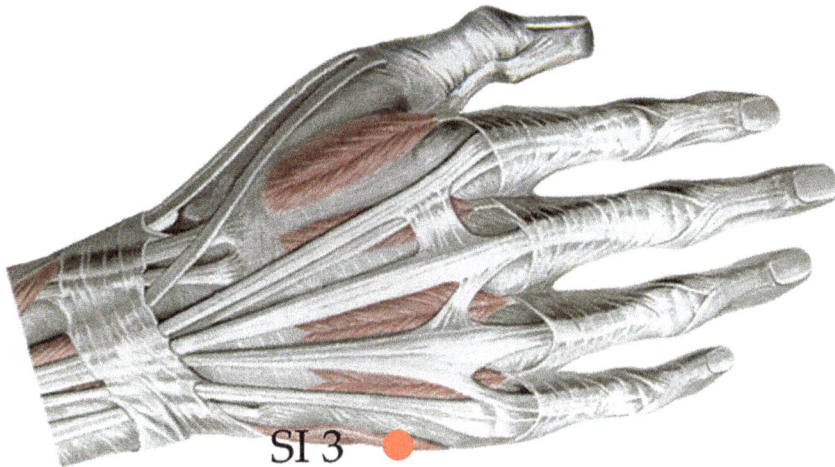

SI 3

SI-5 Yánggǔ — Jing-river point of SI

[Action]	Clears heat and brightens the eyes, calms the spirit and benefits the ears.
[Position]	On the ulnar side of the wrist, in the depression between the styloid process of the ulna and the triangular bone.
[Acupuncture and Moxibustion]	**Acupuncture:** Insert the needle perpendicularly 0.5~0.8 cun deep. **Moxibustion:** Apply 1-3 moxa cones or place a moxa stick above the point for 5~10 minutes.
[Indications]	Headache, pain of the arm and lateral wrist.

SI-8 Xiǎohǎi — He-sea point of SI

[Action]	Clears heat and expels wind, calms the spirit and the heart.
[Position]	On the medial aspect of the elbow, in the depression between the olecranon of the ulna and the medial epicondyle of the humerus.
[Acupuncture and Moxibustion]	**Acupuncture:** Insert the needle perpendicularly 0.2~0.3 cun deep and avoid ulnar nerve: **Moxibustion:** Apply3-5 moxa cones or place a moxa stick above the point for 5~10 minutes.
[Indications]	Headache, psychosis and epilepsy, tinnitus and deafness, pain of the lateral shoulder and arm

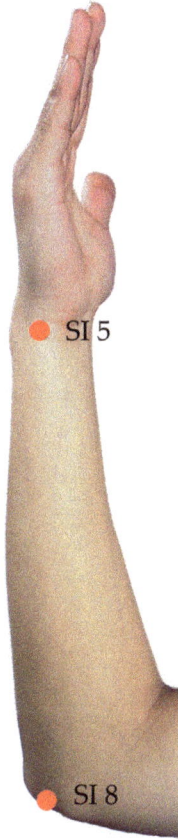

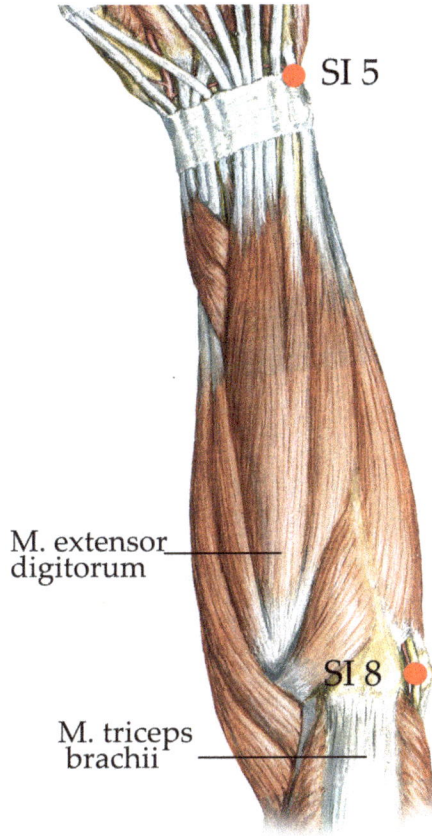

SI 5

SI 5

M. extensor digitorum

SI 8

M. triceps brachii

SI 8

Section VII
Points of Bladder Meridian of Foot Taiyang: BL

BL-67 Zhìyīn — Jing-well point of BL

[Action]	Regulates blood and Qi, turns the fetus and facilitates labour, clears head and eyes.
[Position]	On the lateral border of the end of small toe, 0.1 cun from the lateral corner of the nail.
[Acupuncture and Moxibustion]	**Acupuncture:** Insert the needle subcutaneously 0.1~0.2 cun deep: Or prick with the three-edged needle to bleed. **Moxibustion:** Apply1-3 moxa cones or place a moxa stick above the point for 10~20 minutes.
[Indications]	Mal Position of the fetus and difficult labor.

BL-66 Zútōnggǔ — Ying-spring point of BL

[Action]	Dredges the channel, calms the spirit and benefits intelligence.
[Position]	On the lateral side of the foot, anterior to the fifth. metatarsophalangeal joint, at the junction of the red and white skin.
[Acupuncture and Moxibustion]	**Acupuncture:** Insert the needle perpendicularly 0.2~0.3 cun deep **Moxibustion:** Apply 3-5 moxa cones or place a moxa stick above the point for 5~10 minutes.
[Indications]	Headache, vertigo, psychosis and pain of the toes.

BL-65 Shùgǔ Shu-stream point of BL

[Action]	Dredges the channel and actives the collatrals, clears heat and expels wind.
[Position]	On the lateral side of the foot, posterior to the fifth metatarsophalangeal joint, at the junction of the red and white skin.
[Acupuncture and Moxibustion]	**Acupuncture:** Insert the needle perpendicularly 0.3~0.5 cun deep: **Moxibustion:** Apply 3-5 moxa cones or place a moxa stick above the point for 5~10 minutes.
[Indications]	Headache, red eyes, hemorrhoids and pain in the lateral side of the lower extremities.

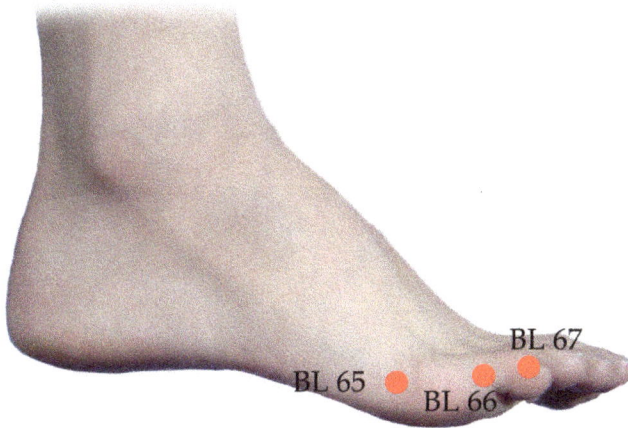

BL 67

BL 65

BL 66

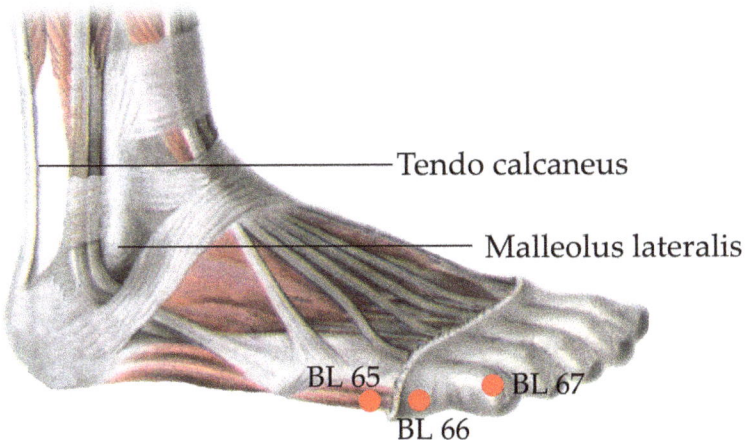

Tendo calcaneus

Malleolus lateralis

BL 65

BL 67

BL 66

BL-60 Kūnlún — Jing-river point of BL

[Action]	Relaxes sinews and activates collaterals, clears head and eyes.
[Position]	On the foot, posterior to the external malleolus, in the depression between the tip of the external malleolus and tendon calcaneus.
[Acupuncture and Moxibustion]	**Acupuncture:** Insert the needle perpendicularly 0.5~1.5 cun deep **Moxibustion:** Apply 5-9 moxa cones or place a moxa stick above the point for 10~20 minutes.
[Indications]	Headache, pain of the waist-and-back.

BL-40 Wěizhōng — He-sea point of BL: lower he-sea point of BL.

[Action]	Clears summer heat, cools blood and detoxify, revives consciousness and calms heart, relaxes sinew and activates collaterals.
[Position]	At the midpoint of the transverse crease of the popliteal fossa, between the tendon of m. biceps femoris and m. semitendinous.
[Acupuncture and Moxibustion]	**Acupuncture:** Insert the needle perpendicularly 0.5~1.0 cun deep: Or prick with a three-edged needle to bleed. **Moxibustion:** Apply 5-7 moxa cones or place a moxa stick above the point for 10~20 minutes.
[Indications]	Lumbar pain, joint pain due to stagnation of damp-cold, weakness of the lower limbs, hemiplegia, beri-beri, erysipelas, boils, furuncle, bruises and spontaneous bleeding under the skin, abdominal pain, vomiting and diarrhea.

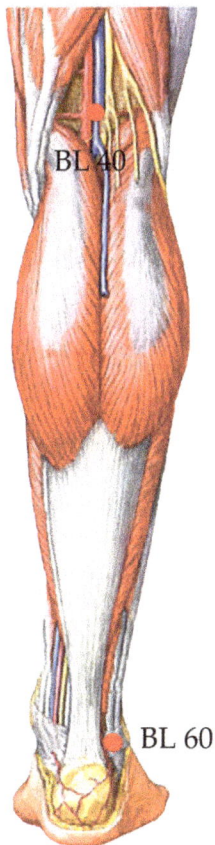 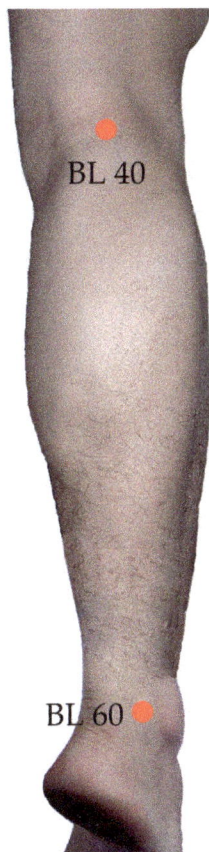

Section VIII
Points of Kidney Merdian of Foot Shaoyin: KI

KI-1 Yǒngquán — Jing-well point of KI

[Action]	Tonifies and nourish kidney, calms liver to extinguish wind, calms spirit and revives consciousness.
[Position]	On the sole of the foot, in the depression when the foot is flexing, on the anterior 1/3 and posterior 2/3 of the sole, on the line connecting the web between the second and the third toes to the back of the heel.
[Acupuncture and Moxibustion]	**Acupuncture:** Insert the needle perpendicularly 0.5~1.0 cun deep: **Moxibustion:** Apply 3-5 moxa cones or place a moxa stick above the point for 5~10 minutes, or use the nature moxibustion.
[Indications]	Fainting, mania, epilepsy, amnesia, panic disorder, infantile convulsion, headache, vertigo, dry tongue, swollen and sore throat, epistaxis, loss of voice, asthma, hemoptysis, consumption, impotence, amenorrhea, protracted labor, infertility, heat in the sole, pain in the all toes, paralysis of the lower limbs and up-rushing gas syndrome.

KI-2 Rángǔ — Ying-spring point of KI

[Action]	Tonifies kidney and nourishes yin, clears heat and eliminates dampness.
[Position]	On the medial side of the foot, below the tuberosity of the navicular bone, at the junction of the red and white skin.
[Acupuncture and Moxibustion]	**Acupuncture:** Insert the needle perpendicularly 0.5~1.0 cun deep. **Moxibustion:** Apply 3-5 moxa cones or place a moxa stick above the point for 5~10 minutes.
[Indications]	Irregular menstruation, distension in the chest and hnypochial.

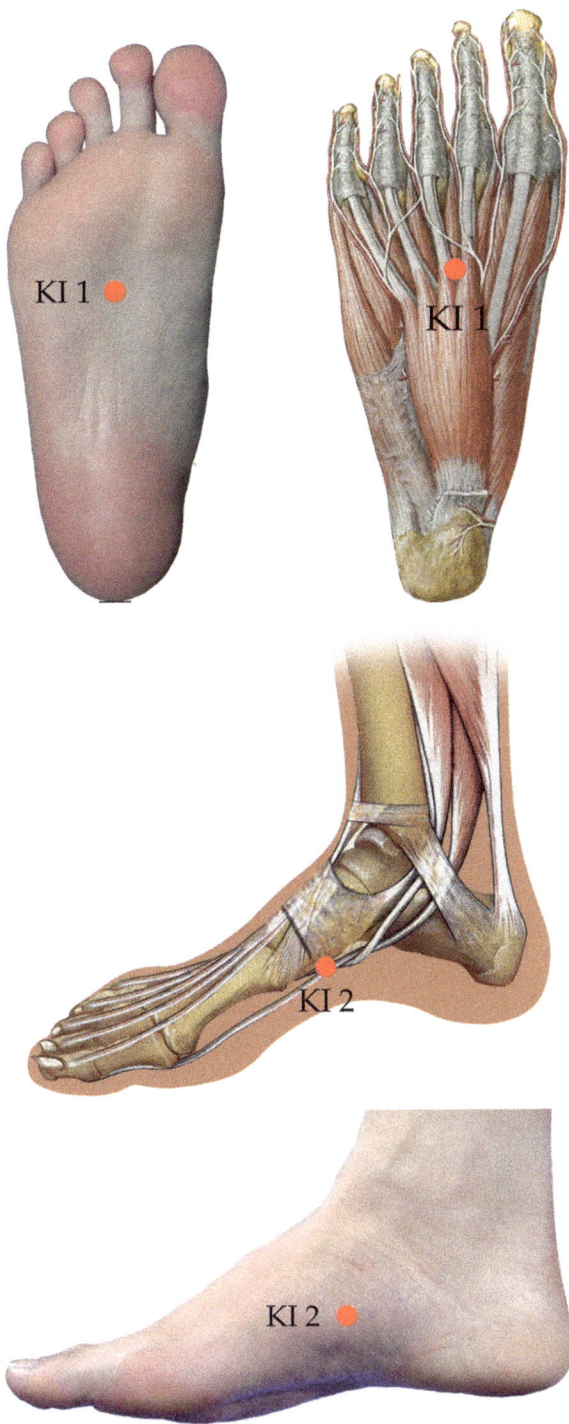

KI 1

KI 1

KI 2

KI 2

KI-3 Tàixī — Shu-stream point of KI

[Action]	Nourishes yin and tonifies kidney, tonifies spleen and benefits lung.
[Position]	On the medial aspect of the foot, in the depression between the tip of the medial malleolus and the tendon calcaneus.
[Acupuncture and Moxibustion]	**Acupuncture:** Insert the needle obliquely 0.5~1.0 cun deep, or there is a numbing and electric sensation radiating to the sole. **Moxibustion:** Apply 3-5 moxa cones or place a moxa stick above the point for 5~10 minutes.
[Indications]	Enuresis, urinary retention, spermatorrhea, impotence, frequent urination, edema, irregular menstruation, amenorrhea, morbid leucorrhea, infertility, cough, asthma, hemoptysis, insomnia, amnesia, neurosis. Headache, toothache, sore throat, sudden loss of voice, epistaxis, tinnitus and deafness, night blindness, soreness and swelling of the internal malleolus and pain of the heel, cold limbs, lumbar pain, consumptive disease, collapse, alopecia and diabetes

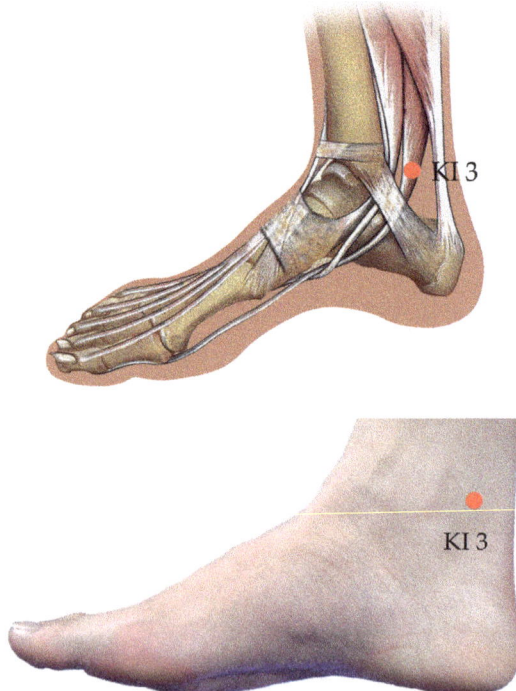

KI 3

KI 3

KI-7 Fùliū — Jing-river point of KI

[Action]	Sweats and relieves exterior syndrome, warms yang to promote diuresis.
[Position]	On the medial aspect of the lower leg, 2 cun directly superior to the tip of the medial ankle, anterior to the tendon calcaneus.
[Acupuncture and Moxibustion]	**Acupuncture:** Insert the needle perpendicularly 0.8~1.0 cun deep **Moxibustion:** Apply 3-5 moxa cones or place a moxa stick above the point for 10~15 minutes.
[Indications]	Edema, abdominal distention, soreness of the waist and spine, swelling of the legs, night sweat, febrile disease without sweating and self-perspiration.

KI-10 Yīngǔ — He-sea point of KI

[Action]	Tonifies kidney and benefits yang, regulates Qi and alleviates pain.
[Position]	In the posterior part of the knee, on the medial aspect of the popliteal stria, lateral to the tendons of m. semitendinusus.
[Acupuncture and Moxibustion]	**Acupuncture:** Insert the needle perpendicularly 0.8~1.2 cun deep **Moxibustion:** Apply 3-5 moxa cones or place a moxa stick above the point for 5~10 minutes.
[Indications]	Spermatorrhea, impotence and irregular menstruation.

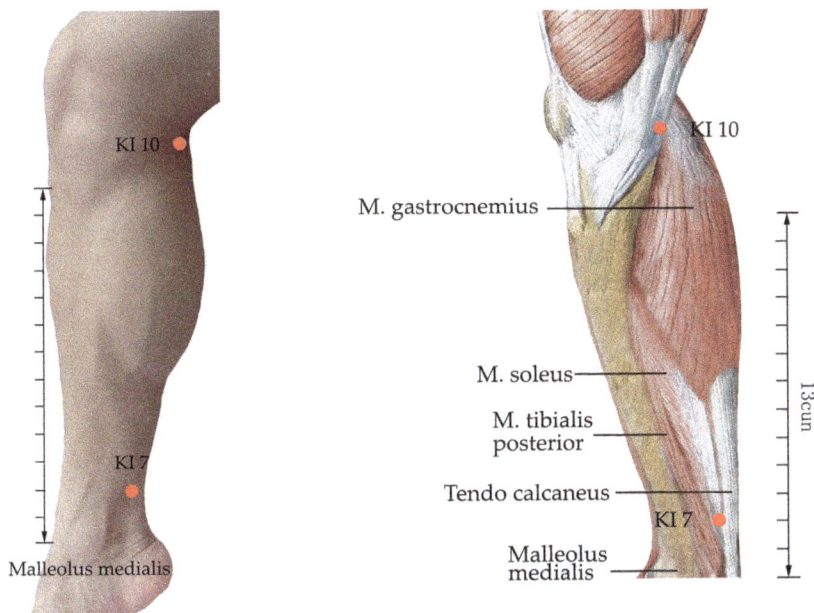

KI 10

M. gastrocnemius

M. soleus

M. tibialis posterior

Tendo calcaneus

KI 7

Malleolus medialis

13cun

Malleolus medialis

Section IX
Points of Pericardium Meridian of Hand Jueyin: PC

PC-9 Zhōngchōng — Jing-well point of PC

[Action]	Rescuing from collapse by restoring yang, revives consciousness and dredges collaterals.
[Position]	In the center of the tip of the distal phalanx of the middle finger.
[Acupuncture and Moxibustion]	**Acupuncture:** Insert the needle subcutaneously 0.1~0.2 cun deep: Or prick with the three-edged needle to bleed. **Moxibustion:** Apply 1-3 moxa cones or place a moxa stick above the point for 5~10 minutes.
[Indications]	Cardiac pain, irritability, stroke, syncope, heatstroke, febrile diseases without sweating and heatstroke, redness of eye, pain of the tongue and night cry during childhood.

PC-8 Láogōng — Ying-spring point of PC

[Action]	Relieves exterior syndrome and restlessness, clears heart heat and revives consciousness.
[Position]	In the center of the palm, between the second and the third metacarpal bones, closer to the third metacarpal bone, when the fist is clenched, under the tip of the third finger.
[Acupuncture and Moxibustion]	**Acupuncture:** Insert the needle perpendicularly 0.3~0.5 cun deep. **Moxibustion:** Apply 1-3 moxa cones or place a moxa stick above the point for 5~10 minutes.
[Indications]	Irritability and anger, laughter, epilepsy and childhood convulsion.

PC 9

PC 8

PC 9

PC 8

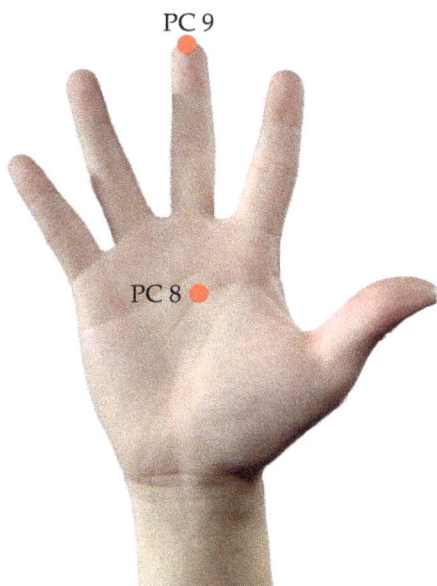

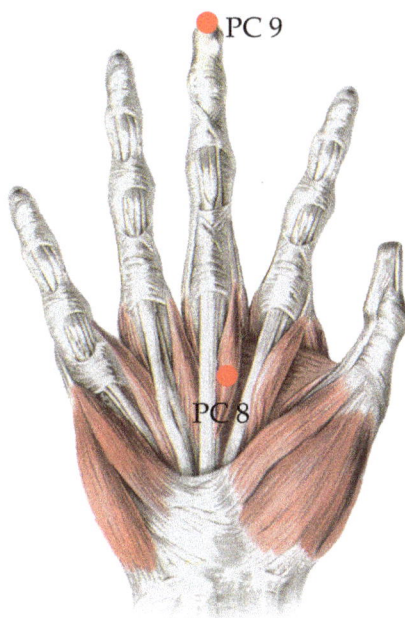

PC-7 Dàlíng — Shu-stream point of PC

[Action]	Clears heart heat and calms spirit, unbinds the chest and harmonizes stomach, dredges channel and activates blood.
[Position]	On the palmar side of the forearm, in the middle of the transverse crease of the wrist, between the tendon of m.palmaris longus and m. flexor carpi radialis.
[Acupuncture and Moxibustion]	**Acupuncture:** Insert the needle perpendicularly 0.3~0.5 cun deep **Moxibustion:** Apply 3-5 moxa cones or place a moxa stick above the point for 10~20 minutes.
[Indications]	Laughter, psychosis, hysteria.

PC-5 Jiānshǐ — Jing-river point of PC

[Action]	Cuts off malaria, unbinds the chest and calms spirit.
[Position]	On the palmar side of the forearm, 3 cun superior to the transverse crease of the wrist, between the tendon of m.palmaris longus and m. flexor carpi radialis.
[Acupuncture and Moxibustion]	**Acupuncture:** Insert the needle perpendicularly 0.5~1.5 cun deep, or until there is a numbing and electric sensation radiating to the finger. **Moxibustion:** Apply 3-7 moxa cones or place a moxa stick above the point for 5~10 minutes.
[Indications]	Malaria, cardiac pain, palpitation, epilepsy, stomach ache and pain of the arm.

PC-3 Qūzé — He-sea point of PC

[Action]	Clears summer heat and benefit heart and Qi, dredges the channel and activates the collaterals, clears heat and detoxifies.
[Position]	On the transverse crease of the elbow, on the ulnar side of the tendon of m. biceps brachii.
[Acupuncture and Moxibustion]	**Acupuncture:** Insert the needle perpendicularly 0.5~1.0 cun deep, and the method is used for treating the diseases of heatstroke, high fever, heat toxin in the blood separation, acute gastroenteritis, and can prick with a three-edged needle to bleed **Moxibustion:** Apply 3-5 moxa cones or place a moxa stick above the point for 5-10 minutes.
[Indications]	Cholera, spasm and pain in the elbow and arm, measles, nettle-rash, heatstroke, fever and acute gastroenteritis.

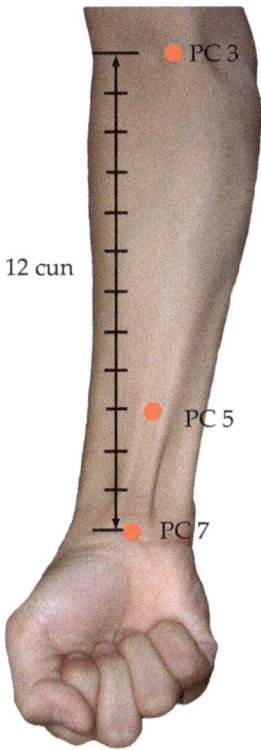

PC 3

12 cun

PC 5

PC 7

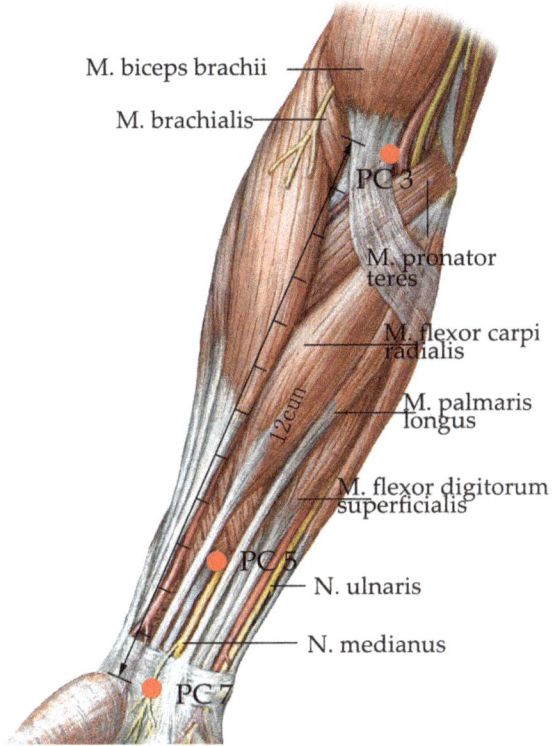

M. biceps brachii

M. brachialis

PC 3

M. pronator teres

M. flexor carpi radialis

M. palmaris longus

M. flexor digitorum superficialis

PC 5

N. ulnaris

N. medianus

PC 7

12 cun

Section X
Points of Sanjiao Meridian of Hand Shaoyang: TE

TE-1 Guānchōng — Jing-well point of TE

[Action]	Clears heat and detoxifies, revives consciousness and dredges the orifices, activates blood and dredges the collaterals.
[Position]	On the ulnar aspect of the distal phalanx of the ring finger, 0.1 cun lateral to the ulnar side of the corner of the nail on the ring finger.
[Acupuncture and Moxibustion]	**Acupuncture:** Insert the needle subcutaneously 0.1~0.3 cun deep: Or prick with the three-edged needle to bleed. **Moxibustion:** Apply 3-5 moxa cones or place a moxa stick above the point for 5~10 minutes.
[Indications]	Headache and febrile diseases without sweating.

TE-2 Yèmén — Xing-spring point of TE

[Action]	Clears heat and calms spirit, dredges collaterals and alleviates pain.
[Position]	On the dorsum aspect of the hand, proximal to the margin of the web between the fourth and fifth finger, at the junction of the red and white skin.
[Acupuncture and Moxibustion]	**Acupuncture:** Insert the needle perpendicularly 0.3~0.5 cun deep **Moxibustion:** Apply 3-5 moxa cones or place a moxa stick above the point for 5~10 minutes.
[Indications]	Febrile diseases without sweating, headache and malaria.

TE-3 Zhōngzhǔ — Shu-stream point of TE

[Action]	Clears heat and dredges the collaterals, benefits the eyes and ears.
[Position]	On the dorsum aspect of the hand, posterior to the fourth metacarpophalangeal joint, in the depression between the fourth and fifth metacarpal bones.
[Acupuncture and Moxibustion]	**Acupuncture:** Insert the needle perpendicularly 0.3~0.5 cun deep **Moxibustion:** Apply 3-5 moxa cones or place a moxa stick above the point for 5~10 minutes.
[Indications]	Deafness, tinnitus, headache and pain of the arm.

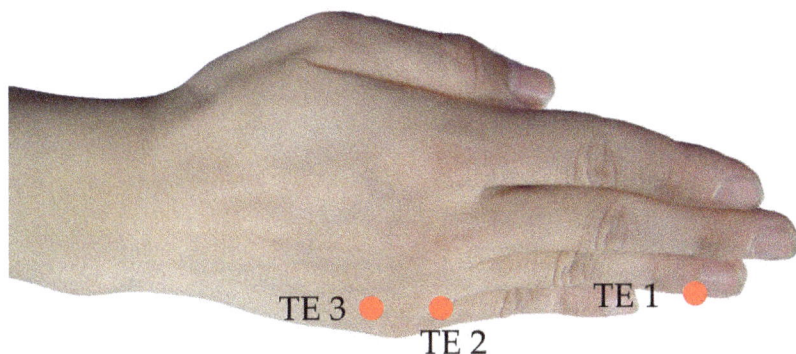

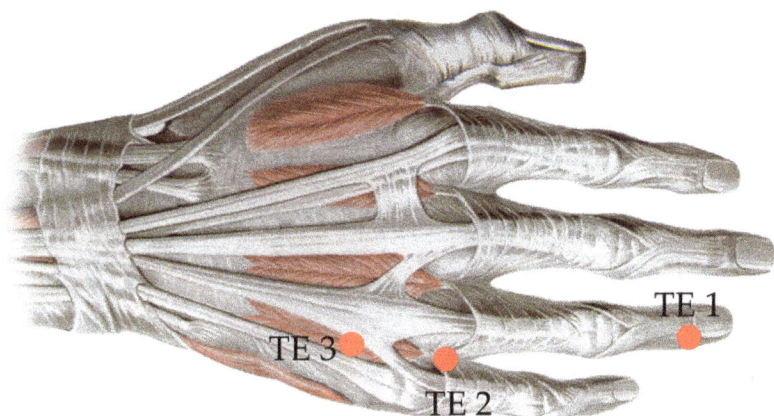

TE-6 Zhīgōu — Jing-river point of TE

[Action]	Expel wind and clears heat, dredges the channel and activates the collaterals.
[Position]	On the dorsal side of the forearm, on the line between SJ 4 (Yangchí) and the tip of the elbow, 3 cun above the transverse crease of the wrist, between the ulna and radius.
[Acupuncture and Moxibustion]	**Acupuncture:** Insert the needle perpendicularly 0.5~1.0 cun deep **Moxibustion:** Apply 3-5 moxa cones or place a moxa stick above the point for 10~20 minutes.
[Indications]	Chest and hypochondriac pain and constipation.

TE-10 Tiānjǐng — He-sea point of TE

[Action]	Regulates Qi and removes stasis, calms spirit and dredges the collaterals.
[Position]	On the lateral side of the arm when the elbow is flexed, in the depression 1 cun proximal to the tip of the elbow.
[Acupuncture and Moxibustion]	**Acupuncture:** Insert the needle perpendicularly 0.5~1.0 cun deep **Moxibustion:** Apply 3-5 moxa cones or place a moxa stick above the point for 10~20 minutes.
[Indications]	Sudden loss of voice, eye disease, scrofula and pain of the arm.

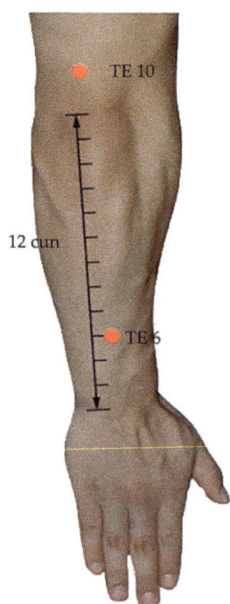

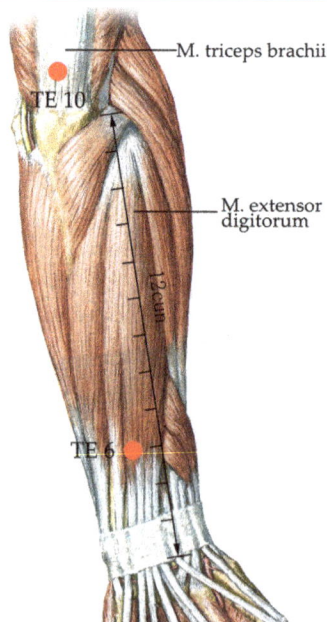

TE 10

12 cun

TE 6

M. triceps brachii

TE 10

M. extensor digitorum

12 cun

TE 6

Section XI
Points of Gallbladder Meridian of Foot Shaoyang: GB

GB-44 Zúqiàoyīn — Jing-well point of GB

[Action]	Clears heat and resolves depression, dredges the channel and activates the collaterals.
[Position]	On the lateral aspect of the fourth toe, 0.1 cun lateral to the corner of the nail.
[Acupuncture and Moxibustion]	**Acupuncture:** Insert the needle subcutaneously 0.1~0.2 cun deep: Or prick with the three-edged needle to bleed. **Moxibustion:** Apply 3-5 moxa cones or place a moxa stick above the point for 5~10 minutes.
[Indications]	Migraine, tinnitus, deafness, redness and pain of the eye, pain of the chest and hypochondrium.

GB-43 Xiáxī — Ying-spring point of GB

[Action]	Clears heat and pacifies wind, reduces swelling and alleviates pain.
[Position]	On the dorsum of the foot, on the margin of the web between the fourth and fifth toes.
[Acupuncture and Moxibustion]	**Acupuncture:** Insert the needle perpendicularly 0.5~0.8 cun deep. **Moxibustion:** Apply 3-5 moxa cones or place a moxa stick above the point for 5~10 minutes.
[Indications]	Headache, tinnitus, deafness, pain of the eye and swollen cheeks.

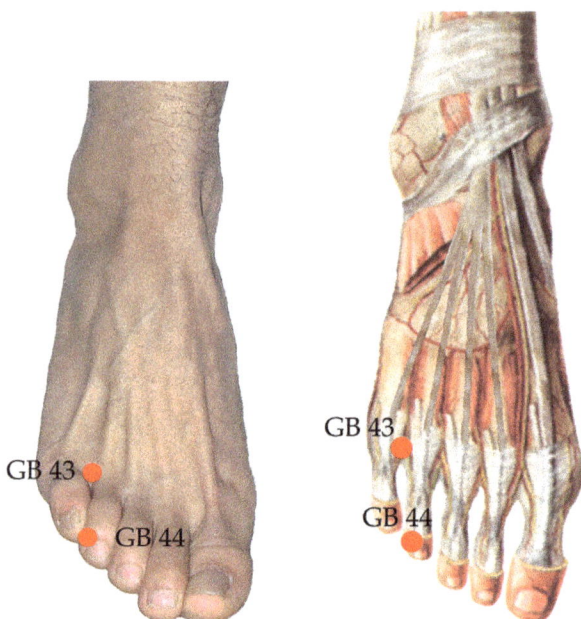

GB 43

GB 43

GB 44

GB 43

GB 44

GB-4 Zúlínqì — Shu-stream point of GB: Confluent point of the girdling vessel

[Action]	Soothing liver-qi stagnation and resolves depression, pacifies wind and clears fire.
[Position]	On the lateral aspect of the dorsum of the foot, distal to the junction of the 4th and 5th metatarsal bone, in the depression on the lateral aspect of the tendon of m. extensor digit minimi of the foot.
[Acupuncture and Moxibustion]	**Acupuncture:** Insert the needle perpendicularly 0.5~0.8 cun deep. **Moxibustion:** Apply 3-5 moxa cones or place a moxa stick above the point for 5~10 minutes.
[Indications]	Headache and dizziness, redness, swelling and pain of the eye, toothache, swollen throat, deafness, mastitis, dyspnea, swelling and pain in the axillary region, pain in the hypochondrium, pain of the knee and ankle and redness and swelling of the dorsum of the foot.

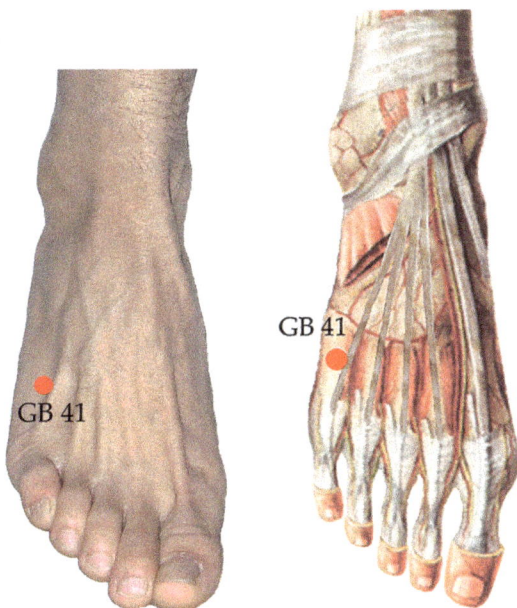

GB 41

GB 41

GB 41

GB-38 Yángfǔ — Jing-river point of GB

[Action]	Expels wind and clears heat, relaxes the sinews and activates the collaterals.
[Position]	On the lateral aspect of the lower leg, 4 cun proximal to the tip of the external malleolus, slightly anterior to the anterior border of the fibula.
[Acupuncture and Moxibustion]	**Acupuncture:** Insert the needle perpendicularly 1.0~1.5 cun deep **Moxibustion:** Apply 3-5 moxa cones or place a moxa stick above the point for 10~20 minutes.
[Indications]	Migraine, pain of the hypochondrium and the chest, pain of the external legs.

GB-34 Yánglíngquán — He-sea point of GB: Influential point of the sinews: Lower he-sea point of GB

[Action]	Clears heat and pacifies wind, relieves swelling and alleviates pain.
[Position]	On the lateral aspect of the lower leg, in the depression anterior and inferior to the head of the fibula.
[Acupuncture and Moxibustion]	**Acupuncture:** Insert the needle perpendicularly towards SP9 (Yīnlíngquán) 1.0~3.0 cun deep **Moxibustion:** Apply 3-5 moxa cones or place a moxa stick above the point for 5~10 minutes.
[Indications]	Headache, tinnitus, deafness, eye pain, swollen cheeks, pain of the chest and hypochondrium, swelling and pain of the breast, asthma, cough, chest distention, vomiting, jaundice, swelling and pain of the knee, weakness and numbness of the lower extremities, spasm, softness, contraction and tightness of the sinews, beriberi and hemiplegia.

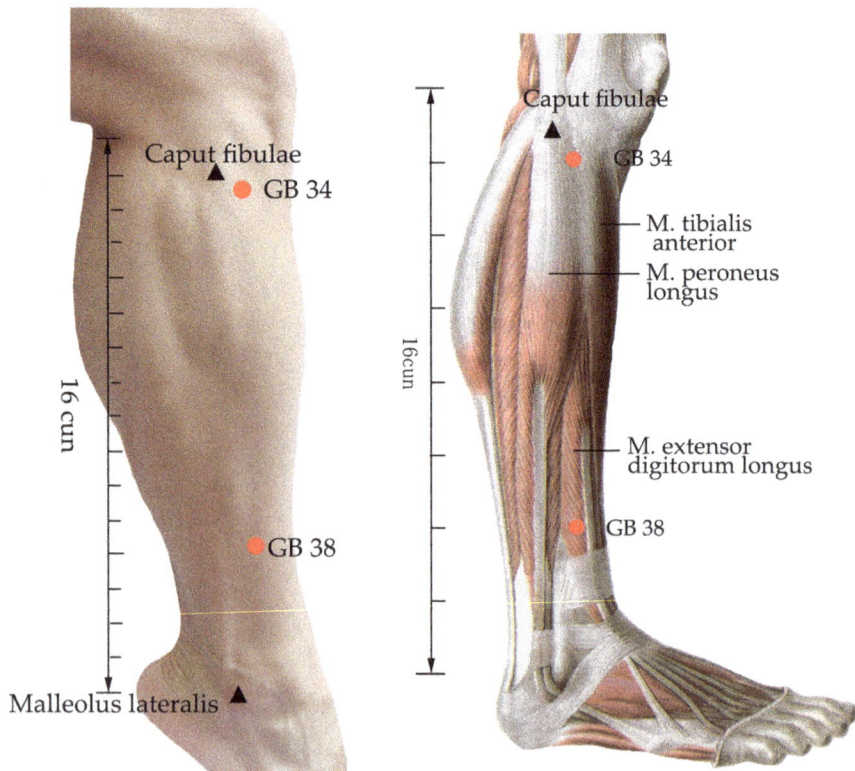

Section XII
Points of Liver Meridian of Foot Jueyin: LR

LR-1 Dàdūn — Jing-well point of LR

[Action]	Regulates Qi and alleviates pain, regulates menstruation and
[Position]	On the foot, 0.1 cun lateral to the corner of the nail of the big toe.
[Acupuncture and Moxibustion]	**Acupuncture:** Insert the needle subcutaneously 0.1~0.2 cun deep: Or prick with the three-edged needle to bleed. **Moxibustion:** Apply 3-5 moxa cones or place a moxa stick above the point for 5~10 minutes.
[Indications]	Amenorrhea, metrorrhagia, prolapsed uterus. hernia, enuresis and disuria.

LR-2 Xíngjiān — Xing-spring point of LR

[Action]	Pacifies liver wind and relaxes the sinews, clears heat and calms spirit, cools blood and stops bleeding.
[Position]	On the dorsum of the foot, proximal to the margin of the web between the first and second toes, at the junction of the red and white skin.
[Acupuncture and Moxibustion]	**Acupuncture:** Insert the needle perpendicularly 0.5~0.8 cun deep **Moxibustion:** Apply 3-5 moxa cones or place a moxa stick above the point for 5~10 minutes.
[Indications]	Headache, vertigo, pain and redness of the eye, tinnitus and deafness, stroke, epilepsy, spermatorrhea, irritability, insomnia, impotence, pruritus vulvae, dysmenorrhea, irregular menstruation.

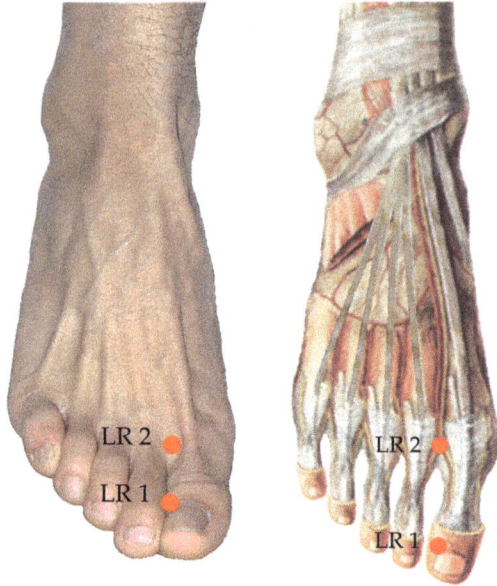

LR-3 Tàichōng — Shu-stream point of LR:Yuan-source point of LR

[Action]	Subdues liver yang and pacifies wind, soothes the liver and nourishes blood.
[Position]	On the dorsum of the foot, between the first and second metatarsal bone, in the depression lateral to the tendon of m. extensor pollicis longus, in the depression proximal to the first metatarsal space.
[Acupuncture and Moxibustion]	**Acupuncture:** Insert the needle perpendicularly 0.5~0.8 cun deep and stimulate until there is a sour, distention or numbing sensation in the local area radiating to the sole of the foot. **Moxibustion:** Apply 3-5 moxa cones or place a moxa stick above the point for 5~10 minutes.
[Indications]	Pain of vulva, enuresis, chest congestion, irregular menstruation, dysmenorrhea, amenorrhea, metrorrhagia, metrostaxis, morbid leucorrhea and mastitis. Infantile convulsions, epilepsy, dizziness, eye pain, headache, irritability and insomnia

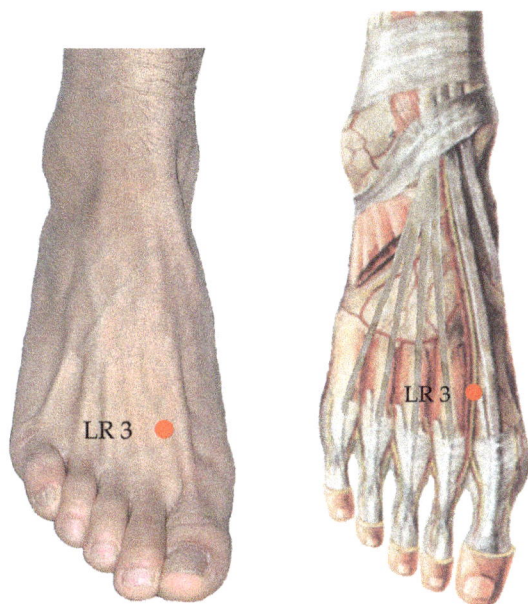

LR-4 Zhōngfēng — Jing-river point of LR

[Action]	Clears liver and gall bladder heat, regulates lower jiao, relaxes sinews and activates the collateral.
[Position]	On the dorsum of the foot, anterior to the medial malleolus, in the depression on the medial border of the tendon.
[Acupuncture and Moxibustion]	**Acupuncture:** Insert the needle perpendicularly 0.5~0.8 cun deep **Moxibustion:** Apply 3-5 moxa cones or place a moxa stick above the point for 5~10 minutes.
[Indications]	Pain and swelling of the medial malleolus, cold of the feet, lower abdominal pain and dry sensation in pharynx.

LR-8 Qūquán — He-sea point of LR

[Action]	Soothing liver-qi stagnation and regulates Qi, regulates menstruation and alleviates pain.
[Position]	On the medial end of the transverse popliteal crease when the knee is flexed, in the depression medial to the m. semitendinosus and m. semimembranosus.
[Acupuncture and Moxibustion]	**Acupuncture:** Insert the needle perpendicularly 1.0~1.5 cun deep **Moxibustion:** Apply 3-5 moxa cones or place a moxa stick above the point for 5~10 minutes.
[Indications]	Impotence, spermatorrhea, prostatitis, irregular menstruation, dysmenorrhea, pruritus vulvae, dysuria and pain of the knee

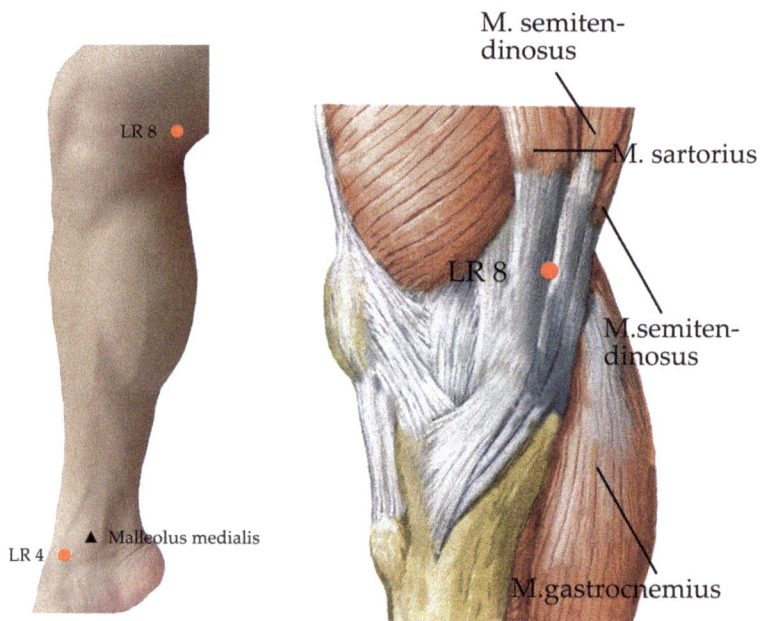

LR 8

LR 4

▲ Malleolus medialis

M. semiten-dinosus

M. sartorius

LR 8

M.semiten-dinosus

M.gastrocnemius

LR 4

CHAPTER 3

Yuan-source Points

LU-9 Tàiyuān — Shu-stream point of LU

[Action]	Alleviates cough and transforms phlegm, regulates and harmonizes the vessels, tonifies Qi and Invigorates the spleen.
[Position]	On the radial end of the wrist crease, in depression ulnar to the m. abductor pollicis longus, between the styloid process of radius and scaphoid bone.
[Acupuncture and Moxibustion]	**Acupuncture:** Insert the needle perpendicularly 0.2~0.3 cun deep. Avoid puncturing the radial artery. **Moxibustion:** Apply 1-3 moxa cones or place a moxa stick above the point for 5-10 minutes.
[Indications]	Cough, asthma, chest congestion, palpitations and pulseless disease.

HT-7 Shénmén — Shu-stream point of HT: Yuan-source point of HT

[Action]	Tonifies the heart and calms the spirit, dredges the channel and actives the collaterals.
[Position]	On the radial side of the tendon m. flexor carpi ulnaris of the transverse wrist crease.
[Acupuncture and Moxibustion]	**Acupuncture:** Insert the needle perpendicularly 0.3~0.5 cun deep and avoid the ulnar artery and vein. **Moxibustion:** Apply 3-5 moxa cones or place a moxa stick above the point for 5~15 minutes.
[Indications]	Irritability, cardiac pain, palpitation, amnesia, insomnia, dementia, psychosis, epilepsy, headache, vertigo, pharyngxerosis, sudden loss of voice, numbness, pain and cold of the arm, asthma, haematemesis and asitia because of the fever.

LU 9

HT 7

A.radialis

Tendo m. flexor
carpi radialis

Tendo m. palmaris
longus

M. flexor carpi ulnaris

LU 9

HT 7

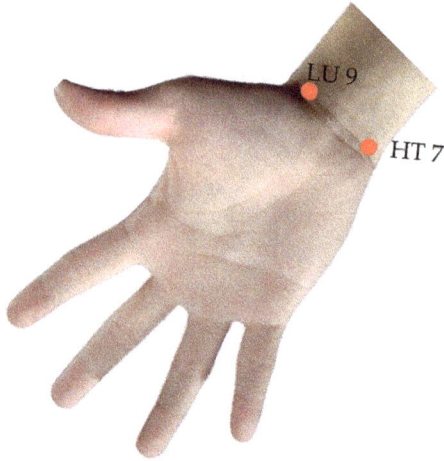

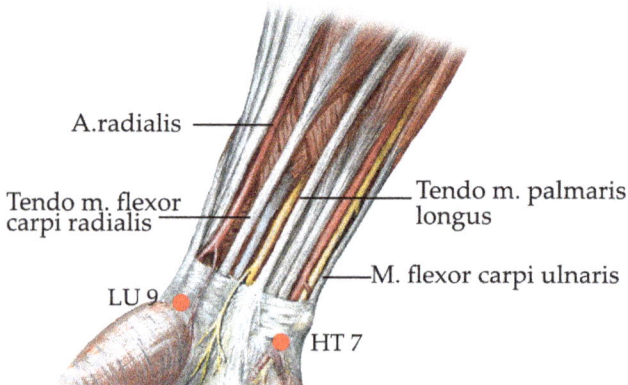

PC-7 Dàlíng — Shu-stream point of PC

[Action]	Clears heart heat and calms spirit, unbinds the chest and harmonizes stomach, dredges channel and activates blood.
[Position]	On the palmar side of the forearm, in the middle of the transverse crease of the wrist, between the tendon of palmaris longus and flexor carpi radialis.
[Acupuncture and Moxibustion]	**Acupuncture:** Insert the needle perpendicularly 0.3~0.5 cun deep: **Moxibustion:** Apply 3-5 moxa cones or place a moxa stick above the point for 10~20 minutes.
[Indications]	Laughter, psychosis, hysteria.

PC 7

A.radialis

Tendo m. flexor
carpi radialis

Tendo m. palmaris
longus

M. flexor carpi ulnaris

PC 7

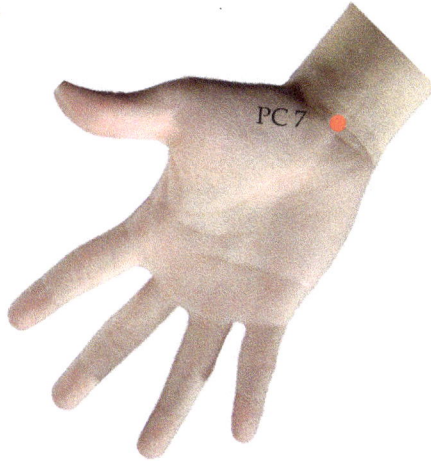

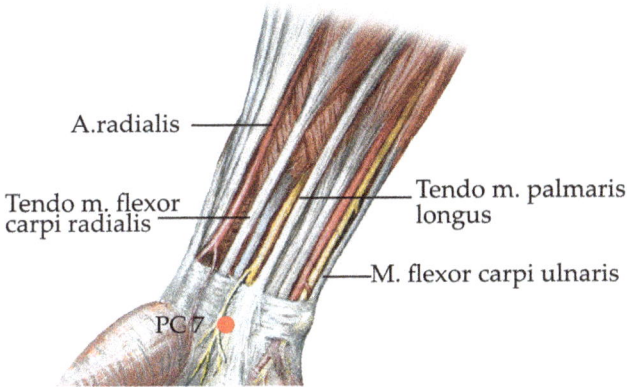

LI-4 Hégǔ — Yuan-source point of LI

[Action]	Calms spirit and alleviates pain, dredges the channel and activates the collaterals, relieves the surface and clears heat.
[Position]	On the dorsum of the hand, between the first and second metacarpal bones, on the radial side of the middle of the second metacarpal bone.
[Acupuncture and Moxibustion]	**Acupuncture:** Insert the needle perpendicularly 0.5~1.0 cun deep
	Moxibustion: Apply 5-7 moxa cones or place a moxa stick above the point for 10~20 minutes. Pregnant women with a history of habitual abortion are not suitable for acupuncture.

[Indications]	Febrile disease without sweat, headache and dizziness, nasal obstruction, epistaxis, rhinorrhea, deafness and tinnitus, redness, swelling and pain of the eye, toothache, mouth ulcers, clenched jaw, deviation of the eye and mouth, soreness of the tongue, stomachache, abdominal pain, constipation, dysentery, irregular menstruation, dysmenorrhea, amenorrhea, protracted labor, excessive excretion of the lochia, retention of the placenta , insufficient lactation, all kinds of pain, addictive rash, skin pruritus, urticaria.

SI-4 Wàngǔ — Yuan-source point of SI

[Action]	Clears damp-heat and treats jaundice, dredges and activates collaterals, increases liquid and eliminates thirst.
[Position]	On the ulnar side of the palm, at the junction of the red and white skin, in the depression between the base of the fifth metacarpal bone and the hamate bone.
[Acupuncture and Moxibustion]	**Acupuncture:** Insert the needle perpendicularly 0.3~0.5 cun deep **Moxibustion:** Apply 3-5 moxa cones or place a moxa stick above the point for 5-10 minutes.
[Indications]	Jaundice, diabetes, headache and stiffness do the neck, pain and spasm of the fingers and arm.

TE-4 Yángchí — Yuan-source point of TE

[Action]	Harmonizes the exterior and the interior, benefits yin and increases liquid.
[Position]	On the dorsum aspect of the transverse wrist crease, in the depression on the ulnar side of the tendon of m. extensor digitorum communis.
[Acupuncture and Moxibustion]	**Acupuncture:** Insert the needle perpendicularly 0.3~0.5 cun deep: **Moxibustion:** Apply 3-5 moxa cones or place a moxa stick above the point for 3~5 minutes.
[Indications]	Diabetes, malaria and redness and swelling of the wrist.

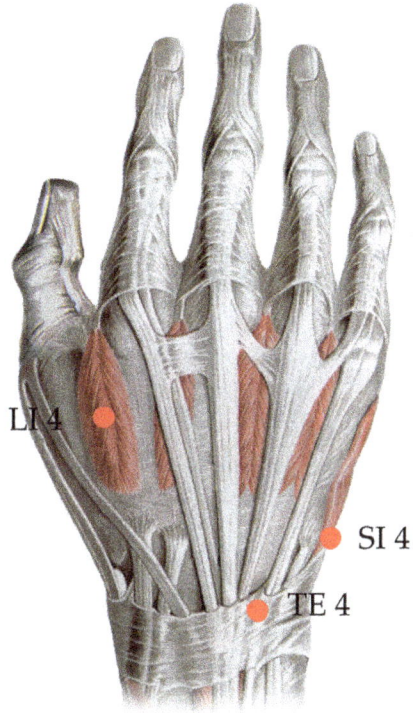

LI 4

SI 4

TE 4

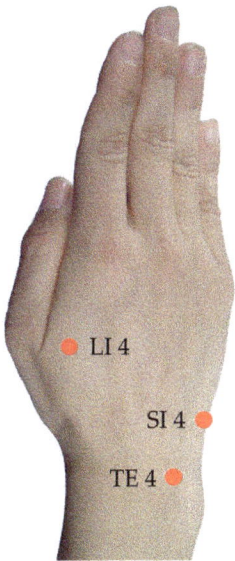

LI 4

SI 4

TE 4

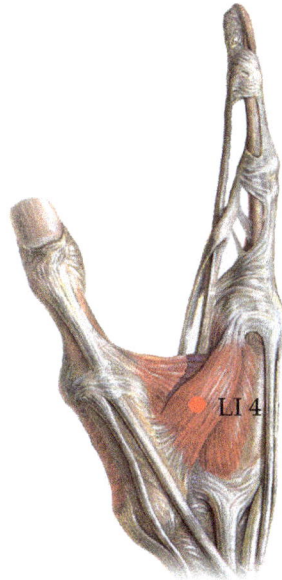

LI 4

SP-3 Tàibái — Yuan-source point of SP:Shu-stream point of SP

[Action]	Invigorates the spleen and harmonizes the stomach, removes dampness and clears heat.
[Position]	On the medial side of foot, in the depression at the junction of red and white skin, posterior and inferior to the proximal metatarsodigital joint of the big toe.
[Acupuncture and Moxibustion]	**Acupuncture:** Insert the needle perpendicularly 0.3~0.5 cun deep **Moxibustion:** Apply1-3 moxa cones or place a moxa stick above the point for 5~10 minutes.
[Indications]	Stomach ache, abdominal distention and pain, borborygmus, vomiting and diarrhea.

KI-3 Tàixī — Yuan-source point of KI:Shu-stream point of KI

[Action]	Nourishes yin and tonifies kidney, tonifies spleen and benefits lung.
[Position]	On the medial aspect of the foot, in the depression between the tip of the medial malleolus and the tendon calcaneus.
[Acupuncture and Moxibustion]	**Acupuncture:** Insert the needle obliquely 0.5~1.0 cun deep, or there is a numbing and electric sensation radiating to the sole. **Moxibustion:** Apply 3-5 moxa cones or place a moxa stick above the point for 5~10 minutes.
[Indications]	Enuresis, urinary retention, spermatorrhea, impotence, frequent urination, edema. Irregular menstruation, amenorrhea, morbid leucorrhea, Infertility, cough, asthma, hemoptysis, insomnia, amnesia, neurosis. Headache, toothache, sore throat, sudden loss of voice, epistaxis, tinnitus and deafness, night blindness, soreness and swelling of the internal malleolus and pain of the heel, cold limbs, lumbar pain, consumptive disease, collapse, alopecia and diabetes.

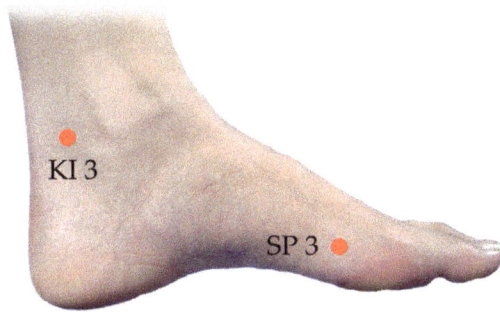

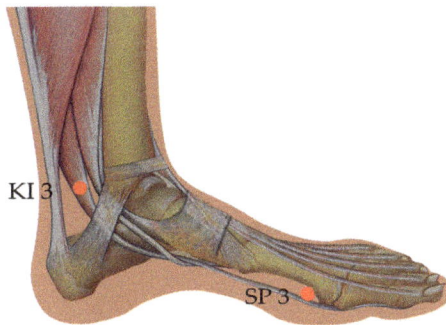

LR-3 Tàichōng — Yuan-source point of LR:Shu-stream point of LR

[Action]	Subdues liver yang and pacifies wind, soothes the liver and nourishes blood.
[Position]	On the dorsum of the foot, between the first and second metatarsal bone, in the depression lateral to the tendon of m.extensor pollicis longus, in the depression proximal to the first metatarsal space.
[Acupuncture and Moxibustion]	**Acupuncture:** Insert the needle perpendicularly 0.5~0.8 cun deep and stimulate until there is a sour, distention or numbing sensation in the local area radiating to the sole of the foot. **Moxibustion:** Apply3-5moxa cones or place a moxa stick above the point for 5~10 minutes.
[Indications]	Pain of vulva, enuresis, chest congestion, irregular menstruation, dysmenorrhea, amenorrhea, metrorrhagia, metrostaxis, morbid leucorrhea and mastitis. Infantile convulsions, epilepsy, dizziness, pain of the eye, headache, irritability and insomnia.

ST-42 Chōngyáng — Yuan-source point of ST

[Action]	Harmonizes the stomach and transforms phlegm, dredges the collaterals and calms the spirit.
[Position]	On the dorsum of the foot, between the extensor pollicis longus muscle tendon and extensor digitorum longus where the pulse of the dorsal artery can be felt.
[Acupuncture and Moxibustion]	**Acupuncture:** Avoid puncturing the artery and insert the needle perpendicularly 0.2~0.3 cun deep. **Moxibustion:** Apply 3-5 moxa cones or place a moxa stick above the point for 5~10 minutes.
[Indications]	Stomach ache, abdominal distention, paralysis of the foot, swelling and pain of the dorsum of the foot, manic psychosis.

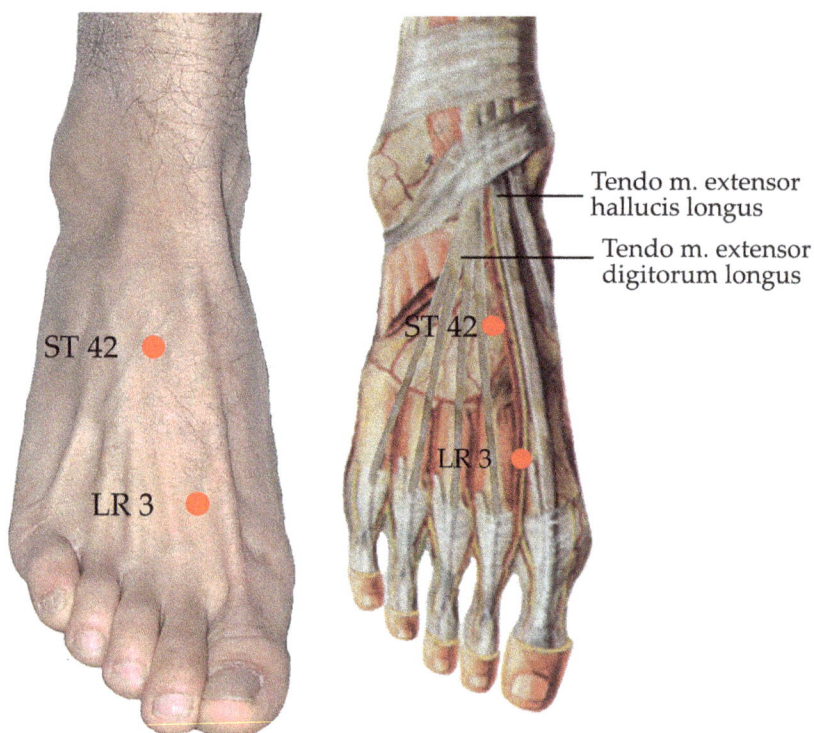

Tendo m. extensor hallucis longus

Tendo m. extensor digitorum longus

ST 42

LR 3

BL-64 Jīnggǔ — Yuan-source point of BL

[Action]	Clears heat and expels wind, regulates heart and calms spirit.
[Position]	On the lateral side of the foot, inferior to the tuberosity of the fifth metatarsal bone, at the junction of the red and white skin.
[Acupuncture and Moxibustion]	**Acupuncture:** Insert the needle perpendicularly 0.3~0.5 cun deep **Moxibustion:** Apply3-7 moxa cones or place a moxa stick above the point for 5-10 minutes.
[Indications]	Headache, vertigo, stiff neck and lumbago.

GB-40 Qiūxū — Yuan-source point of GB

[Action]	Clears summer heat, cools blood and removes toxins, revives consciousness and calms spirit, relaxes sinews and activates the collaterals.
[Position]	Anterior and inferior to the external malleolus, in the depression on the lateral aspect of the tendon of m. extensor digitorum longus.
[Acupuncture and Moxibustion]	**Acupuncture:** Insert the needle perpendicularly 0.5~1.0 cun deep. **Moxibustion:** Apply 5-7 moxa cones or place a moxa stick above the point for 10-20 minutes.
[Indications]	Migraine, pain of the chest and hypochondrium, aches of the legs and lumbago and malaria.

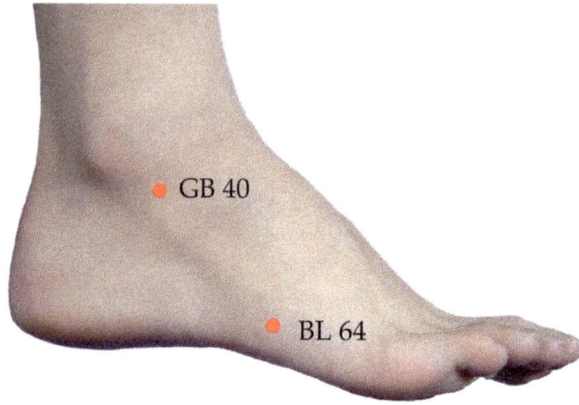

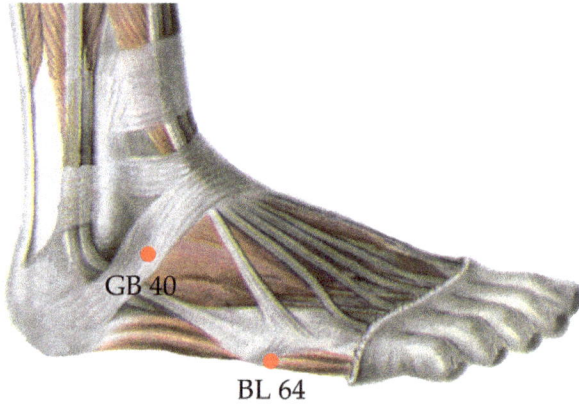

CHAPTER 4

Luo-connecting Points

LU-7 Lièquē — Luo-connecting point of LU: Confluent points of the Ren vessel

[Action]	Releases the exterior and expels wind, regulates the Ren vessel.
[Position]	On the radial side of the forearm, 1.5 cun proximal the transverse crease of the wrist, superior to the styolid process of the radius and between tendons of m. bra-chioradialis and m. abductor pollicis longus.
[Acupuncture and Moxibustion]	**Acupuncture:** Insert the needle obliquely upward 0.2~0.3 cun deep. **Moxibustion:** Apply 3-5 moxa cones or place a moxa stick above the point for 5~10 minutes.
[Indications]	Cough, asthma, shortness of breath, headache and migraine, neck stiffness and sore throat,

HT-5 Tōnglǐ — Luo-connecting point of HT

[Action]	Calms the spirit, clears deficient heat, dredges the channel and activates the collaterals.
[Position]	On the palmar aspect of the forearm, on the radial aspect of the tendon m. flexor carpi ulnaris, 1 cun proximal to the transverse wrist crease.
[Acupuncture and Moxibustion]	**Acupuncture:** Insert the needle perpendicularly 0.3~0.5 cun deep **Moxibustion:** Apply 1-3 moxa cones or place a moxa stick above the point for 10~20 minutes.
[Indications]	Cardiac pain, headache, vertigo and night sweat.

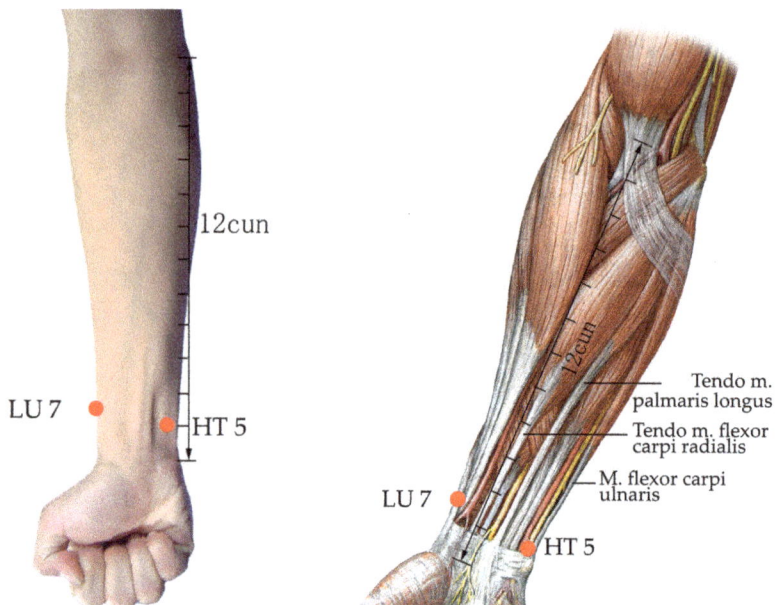

12cun

LU 7

HT 5

Tendo m. palmaris longus
Tendo m. flexor carpi radialis
M. flexor carpi ulnaris

LU 7

HT 5

PC 6 Nèiguān — Luo-connecting point of PC; Confluent point of the yin linking vessel

[Action]	Regulates heart and calms the spirit, descends rebellious Qi and regulates stomach, unbinds the chest and regulates Qi, clears heat and alleviates pain.
[Position]	On the palmar aspect of the forearm, 2 cun superior to the transverse crease of the wrist, between the tendon of m.palmaris longus and m. flexor carpi radialis.
[Acupuncture and Moxibustion]	**Acupuncture:** Insert the needle perpendicularly 0.5~1.5 cun deep. **Moxibustion:** Apply 5-7 moxa cones or place a moxa stick above the point for 10~20 minutes.
[Indications]	Cardiac pain, palpitation, insomnia, stomachache, vomiting, hiccough and asthma.

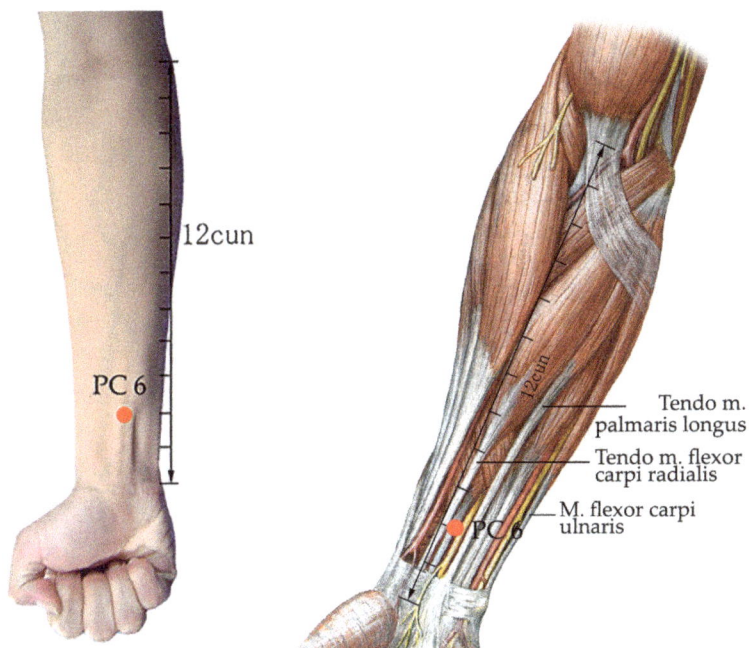

12cun

PC 6

12cun

Tendo m. palmaris longus

Tendo m. flexor carpi radialis

M. flexor carpi ulnaris

PC 6

LI-6 Piānlì — Luo-connecting point of LI

[Action]	Clears heat and induces diuresis, dredges the channel and activates the collaterals.
[Position]	On the radial side of the back of the forearm, 3 cun proximal to the wrist crease, in the line connecting LI 5 (Yáng xī) and LI 11 (Qǔchí) when the elbow is flexed.
[Acupuncture and Moxibustion]	**Acupuncture:** Insert the needle perpendicularly 0.3~0.5 cun deep. **Moxibustion:** Apply 3-5 moxa cones or needle-warming moxibustion or place a moxa stick above the point for 5~10 minutes.
[Indications]	Deafness, tinnitus, epistaxis, borborygums and abdominal pain.

SI-7 Zhīzhèng — Luo-connecting point of SI

[Action]	Clears heat and removes toxicity, calms the spirit, dredges the channel and activates the collaterals.
[Position]	On the anterior border of the ulnar, on the line connecting SI 5 (yáng gǔ) to SI 8 (xiǎo hǎi), 5 cun pdroximal to the posterior transverse wrist crease, in the depression between the ulnar side of the ulna and m. flexor carpi ulnaris.
[Acupuncture and Moxibustion]	**Acupuncture:** Insert the needle perpendicularly or obliquely 0.5~1.0 cun deep. **Moxibustion:** Apply 3-5 moxa cones or needle-warming moxibustion or place a moxa stick above the point for 5~10 minutes.
[Indications]	Aches of the back and waist, weakness of limbs.

TE-5 Wàiguān — Luo-connecting point of TE: Confluent points of the yang linking vessel

[Action]	Clears heat and releases exterior, dredges the channel and activates the collaterals.
[Position]	On the dorsal side of the forearm, 2 cun proximal to the transverse crease of the wrist, in the depression between the ulna and radius.
[Acupuncture and Moxibustion]	**Acupuncture:** Insert the needle perpendicularly or obliquely 0.5~1.0 cun deep. **Moxibustion:** Apply 3-5 moxa cones or needle-warming moxibustion or place a moxa stick above the point for 10~20 minutes.
[Indications]	Febrile diseases, common cold, headache, tinnitus, chest and hypochondriac pain, inability to raise arm.

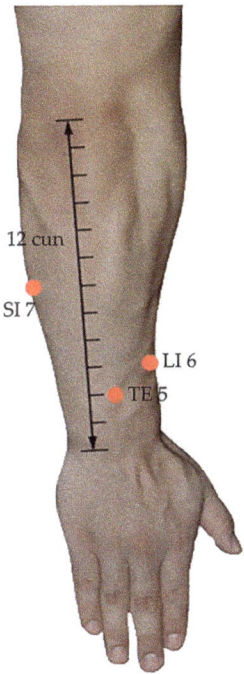

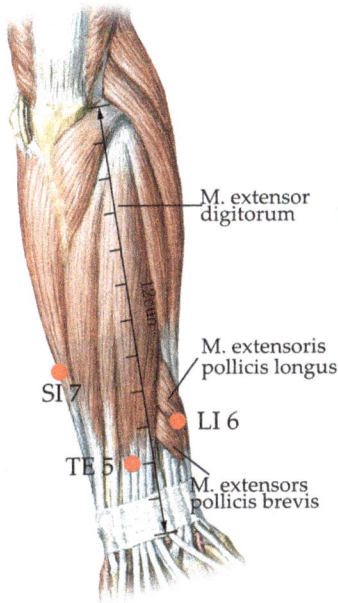

12 cun

SI 7

LI 6

TE 5

M. extensor digitorum

M. extensoris pollicis longus

SI 7

LI 6

TE 5

M. extensors pollicis brevis

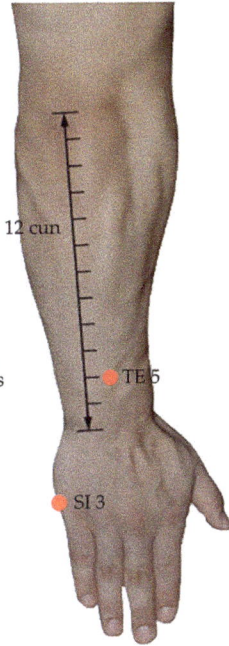

12 cun

TE 5

SI 3

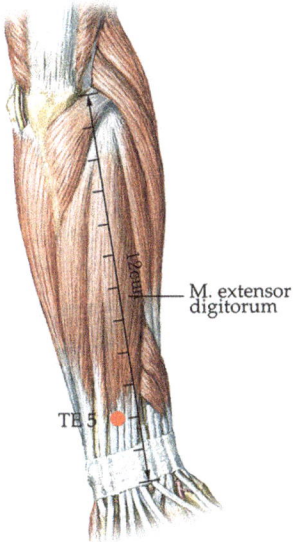

M. extensor digitorum

TE 5

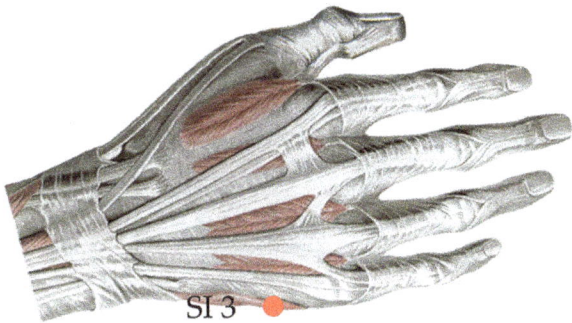

SI 3

LR-5 Lígōu — Luo-connecting point of LV

[Action]	Soothing liver-qi stagnation and regulates Qi, regulates menstruation and leucorrhea.
[Position]	On the medial aspect of the lower limb, 5 cun proximal to the tip of the medial malleolus, in the center of the medial aspect of the tibia.
[Acupuncture and Moxibustion]	**Acupuncture:** Insert the needle perpendicularly 1.0~1.2 cun deep. **Moxibustion:** Apply 3-5 moxa cones or needle-warming moxibustion or place a moxa stick above the point for 10~20 minutes.
[Indications]	Hernia, enuresis, urinary retention, irregular menstruation, bloody and morbid leucorrhea, prolapse of the uterus, metrorrhagia and metrostaxis.

SP-4 Gōngsūn — Luo-connecting point of SP; Confluent point of the Chong vessel

[Action]	Invigorates the spleen and stomach, regulates the Chong vessels and Ren vessels.
[Position]	On the medial side of the foot, in the depression anterior and inferior to the base of the first metatarsal bone, at the junction of the red and white skin.
[Acupuncture and Moxibustion]	**Acupuncture:** Insert the needle perpendicularly 0.5~0.8 cun deep. **Moxibustion:** Apply 3-5 moxa cones or place a moxa stick above the point for 10-20 minutes.
[Indications]	Vomiting, abdominal pain, stomach ache, borborygums, diarrhea and dysentery.

KI-4 Dàzhōng — Luo-connecting point of KI

[Action]	Induces diuresis for removing edema, tonifies kidney and regulates menstruation, clears heat and calms spirit.
[Position]	On the medial side of the foot, posterior and inferior to the medial malleous, in the depression anterior to the anterior border of the tendon calcaneus.

[Acupuncture and Moxibustion]	Acupuncture: Insert the needle perpendicularly 0.5~1.0 cun deep Moxibustion: Apply 3-5 moxa cones or place a moxa stick above the point for 5~10 minutes.
[Indications]	Swelling and pain of the throat and stiffness and pain of the lumbago.

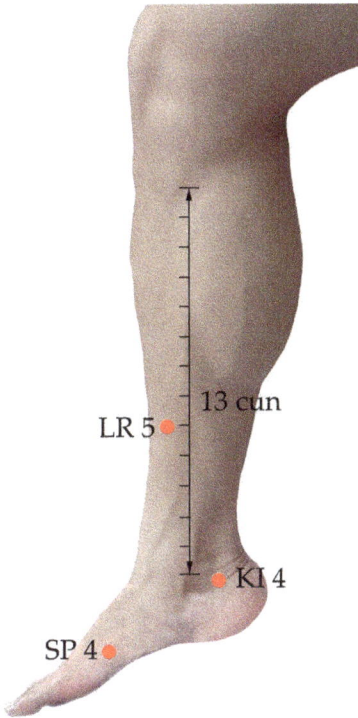

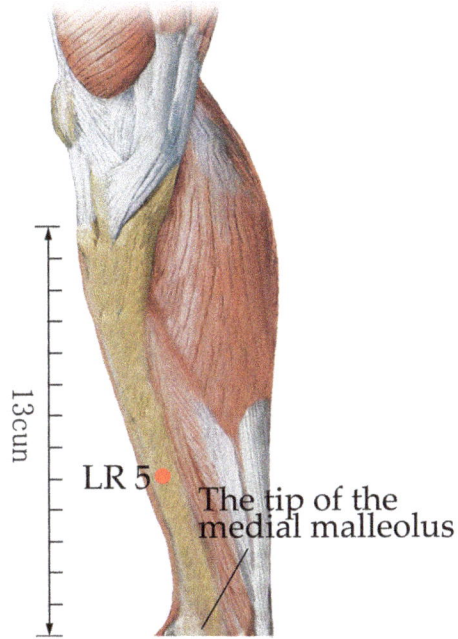

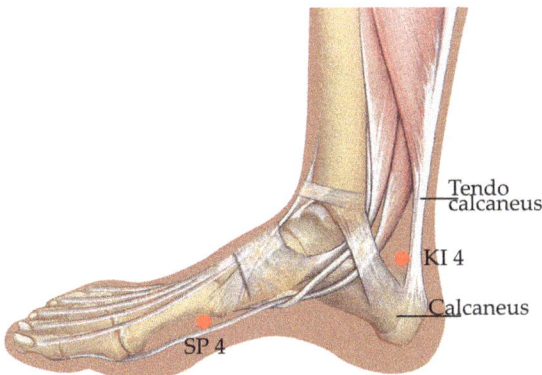

13 cun

LR 5

KI 4

SP 4

13cun

LR 5

The tip of the medial malleolus

Tendo calcaneus

KI 4

Calcaneus

SP 4

ST-40 Fēnglóng — Luo-connecting point of ST

[Action]	Invigorates the spleen and dissipates phlegm, harmonizes stomach and lowers adverse Qi.
[Position]	On the anterior and lateral aspect of the leg, 8 cun superior to the tip of the lateral malleolus, two finger width lateral from the anterior ridge of the tibia.
[Acupuncture and Moxibustion]	**Acupuncture:** Insert the needle perpendicularly 1.0~1.5 cun deep **Moxibustion:** Apply 5-7 moxa cones or place a moxa stick above the point for 10~20 minutes.
[Indications]	Stupum, stomachache, constipation, psychosis, epilepsy, somnolence, hysteria, globus hysteriocus, choking cough, asthma.

BL-58 Fēiyáng — Luo-connecting point of BL

[Action]	Relaxes sinews and activates collaterals, clears heat and removes swelling.
[Position]	On the posterior side of the lower leg, 7 cun superior to BL 60 (Kūnlún), between the inferior and lateral margin of the gastrocnmius and heel tendon.
[Acupuncture and Moxibustion]	**Acupuncture:** Insert the needle perpendicularly 0.7~1.0 cun deep. **Moxibustion:** Apply 3-5 moxa cones or needle-warming moxibustion or place a moxa stick above the point for 5~10 minutes.
[Indications]	Pain of the leg and waist, weakness of the knees and aches of the legs.

GB-37 Guāngmíng — Luo-connecting point of GB

[Action]	Soothing liver-qi stagnation and benefits the eyes, dredges the channel and activates the collaterals.
[Position]	On the lateral aspect of the lower leg, 5 cun proximal to the tip of the external malleolus, on the anterior border of the fibula.
[Acupuncture and Moxibustion]	**Acupuncture:** Insert the needle perpendicularly 1.0~1.2 cun deep. **Moxibustion:** Apply 3-5 moxa cones or needle-warming moxibustion or place a moxa stick above the point for 10~20 minutes.
[Indications]	Redness, swelling and pain of the eye, blurred vision, mastitis, atrophy and paralysis of the lower limbs.

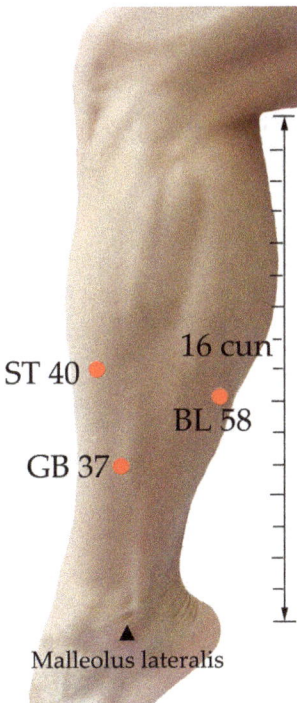

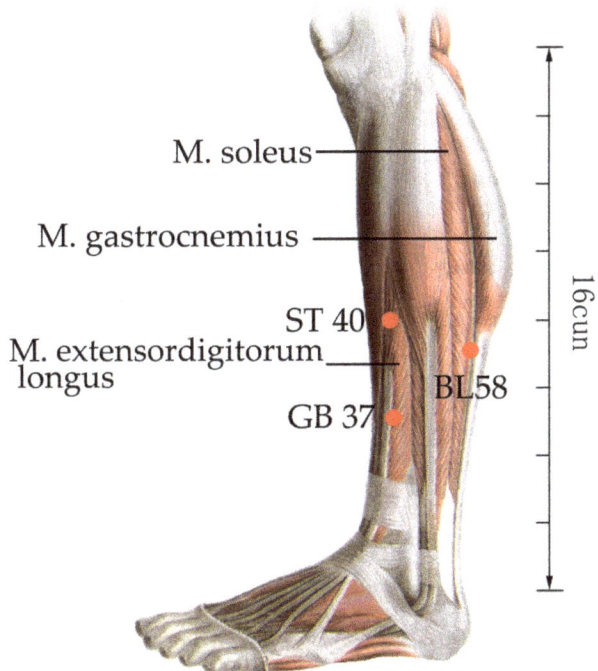

RN-15 Jiūwěi — Luo-connecting point of RN

[Action]	Unbinds the chest and harmonizes the diaphragm, regulates heart and calms spirit.
[Position]	On the upper abdomen, on the anterior midline, 1 cun inferior to the sternocostal angle.
[Acupuncture and Moxibustion]	**Acupuncture:** Insert the needle obliquely downwards 0.3~0.5 cun deep and avoid deep puncture to prevent injury to the heart and the liver. **Moxibustion:** Apply 3-5 moxa cones or place a moxa stick above the point for 10~20 minutes.
[Indications]	Chest distention and cough.

SP-21 Dàbāo — Great luo-connecting point of SP

[Action]	Unbinds the chest and invigorates spleen, regulates Qi and blood.
[Position]	On the lateral aspect of the chest, on the mid-axillary line, 6 cun inferior to the center of the axilla, in the sixth intercostal space.
[Acupuncture and Moxibustion]	**Acupuncture:** Insert the needle obliquely towards the spine 0.5~0.8 cun deep. **Moxibustion:** Apply 3 moxa cones or place a moxa stick above the point for 10~20 minutes or natural moxibustion.
[Indications]	Pain of the chest and hypochondriac region, asthma, cough and weakness of the limbs.

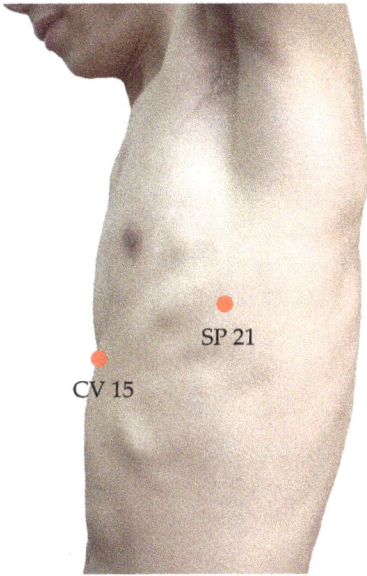

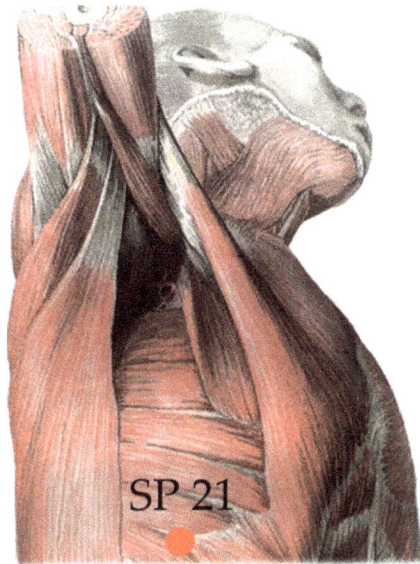

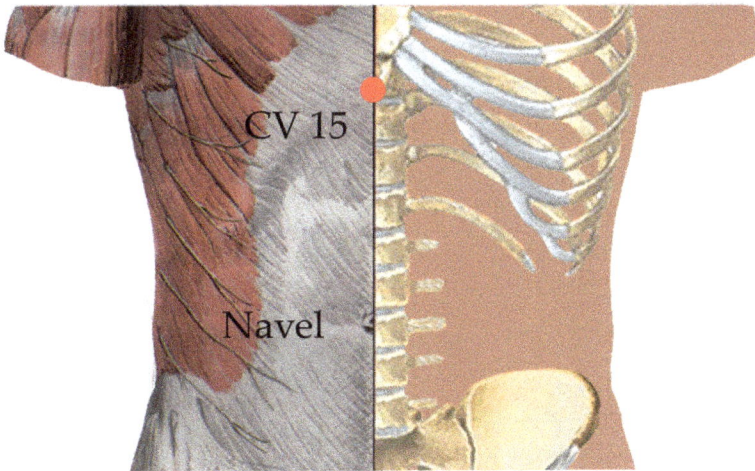

GV-1 Chángqiáng — Luo-connecting point of DU

[Action]	Nourishes yin and descents yang, nourishes Qi to stop collapse.
[Position]	Below the tip of the coccyx, at the midpoint between the tip of the coccyx and the anus.
[Acupuncture and Moxibustion]	**Acupuncture:** Insert the needle obliquely upwards 0.5~1.0 cun deep proximally to the anterior border of the coccyx. Prick with the three-edged needle to bleed. **Moxibustion:** Moxibustion is prohibited.
[Indications]	Diarrhea, constipation, blood in the stool, hemorrhoids and prolapsus of the rectum.

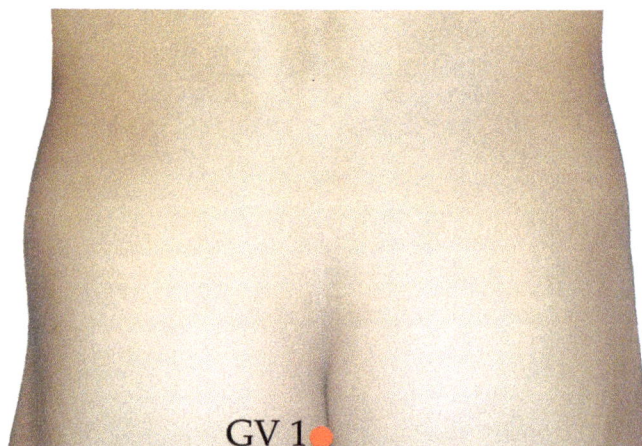

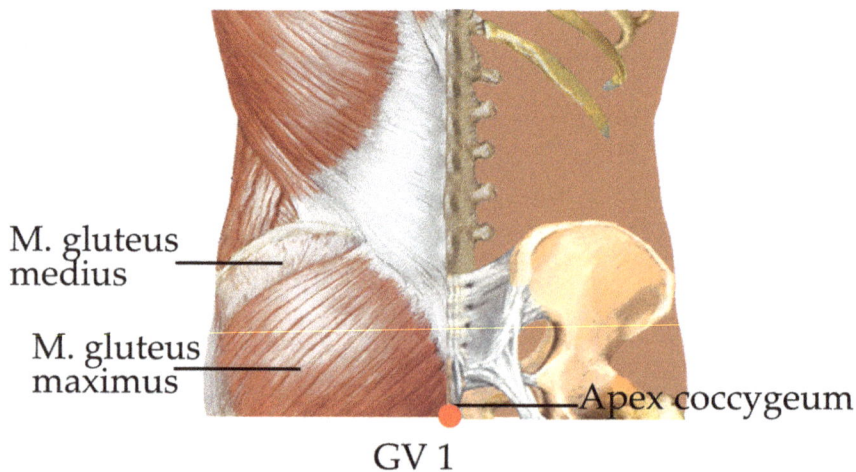

GV 1

M. gluteus medius

M. gluteus maximus

Apex coccygeum

GV 1

CHAPTER 5

Back-shu Points

BL-13 Fèishū — Back-shu point of LU

[Action]	Clears heat and releases the exterior, descends and disperses lung Qi.
[Position]	On the upper back, 1.5 cun lateral to the lower border of the spinous process of the third thoracic vertebra.
[Acupuncture and Moxibustion]	**Acupuncture:** Insert the needle obliquely towards the spine 0.5~0.8 cun deep. **Moxibustion:** Apply 5-9 moxa cones or place a moxa stick above the point for 10~20 minutes or natural moxibustion.
[Indications]	Cough, chest distention and asthma, urticaria, back pain.

BL-14 Juéyīnshū — Back-shu point of PC

[Action]	Activates blood and regulates Qi, clears heart and calms spirit.
[Position]	On the upper back, 1.5 cun lateral to the lower border of the spinous process of the fourth thoracic vertebra.
[Acupuncture and Moxibustion]	**Acupuncture:** Insert the needle obliquely towards the spine 0.5~0.8 cun deep. **Moxibustion:** Apply 5-9 moxa cones or place a moxa stick above the point for 10~20 minutes.
[Indications]	Cardiac pain, palpitation and chest distention.

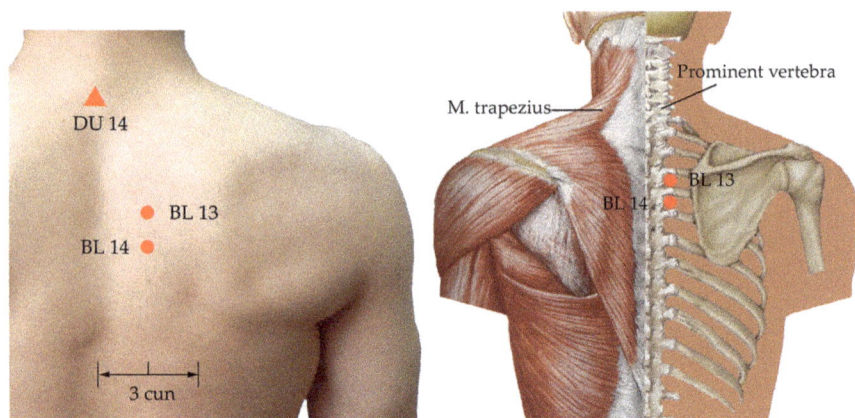

Prominent vertebra

M. trapezius

DU 14

BL 13

BL 14

BL 13

BL 14

3 cun

BL-15 Xīnshū — Back-shu point of HT

[Action]	Regulates Qi and blood, dredges heart and collaterals and calms heart.
[Position]	On the upper back, 1.5 cun lateral to the lower border of the spinous process of the fifth thoracic vertebra.
[Acupuncture and Moxibustion]	**Acupuncture:** Insert the needle obliquely towards the spine 0.5~0.8 cun deep. **Moxibustion:** Apply 5-9 moxa cones or place a moxa stick above the point for 10~20 minutes or natural moxibustion.
[Indications]	Pain on the chest, shoulder and back, cardiac pain, palpitation, chest distention, mania, epilepsy, psychosis, insomnia, amnesia, nocturnal emission, night sweat.

BL-18 Gānshū — Back-shu point of LV

[Action]	Soothing liver-qi stagnation liver and regulates Qi, clears gallbladder and removes depression.
[Position]	On the back, 1.5 cun lateral to the lower border of the spinous process of the ninth thoracic vertebra.
[Acupuncture and Moxibustion]	**Acupuncture:** Insert the needle obliquely towards the spine 0.5~0.8 cun deep. **Moxibustion:** Apply 5-9 moxa cones or place a moxa stick above the point for 10~20 minutes.
[Indications]	Abdominal distention, chest congestion, jaundice, vomiting, mania, psychosis and epilepsy, dizziness, pain and eye redness, eye diseases, cold hernia and irregular menstruation.

BL 19 Dǎnshū — Back-shu point of GB

[Action]	Sooths liver-Qi stagnation liver and clears gallbladder, clears heat and nourishes yin, harmonizes the stomach and descends Qi.
[Position]	On the back, 1.5 cun lateral to the lower border of the spinous process of the tenth thoracic vertebra.
[Acupuncture and Moxibustion]	**Acupuncture:** Insert the needle obliquely towards the spine 0.5~0.8 cun deep. **Moxibustion:** Apply 5-9 moxa cones or place a moxa stick above the point for 10~20 minutes.
[Indications]	Jaundice, pain in the chest and hypochondriac region, Stomach ache, vomiting, tuberculosis.

BL-20 Píshū — Back-shu point of SP

[Action]	Invigorates spleen Qi to control the blood, harmonizes stomach and benefits Qi.
[Position]	On the back, 1.5 cun lateral to the lower border of the spinous process of the eleventh thoracic vertebra.
[Acupuncture and Moxibustion]	**Acupuncture:** Insert the needle obliquely towards the spine 0.5~0. 8 cun deep. **Moxibustion:** Apply 5-9 moxa cones or place a moxa stick above the point for 10~20 minutes.
[Indications]	Abdominal distention, vomiting, diarrhea, dysentery, Stomach ache, gluten, blood in urine, diabetes.

BL-21 Wèishū — Back-shu point of ST

[Action]	Invigorates the spleen and harmonizes stomach: resolves dampness (the state of body feeling damp) and promotes digestion.
[Position]	On the back, 1.5 cun lateral to the lower border of the spinous process of the twelfth thoracic vertebra.
[Acupuncture and Moxibustion]	**Acupuncture:** Insert the needle perpendicularly 0.8~1.0 cun deep. **Moxibustion:** Apply 5-9 moxa cones or place a moxa stick above the point for 10~20 minutes.
[Indications]	Stomach ache, nausea, vomiting, borborygmus diarrhea,

3 cun

DU 9

BL 19
BL 20
BL 21

BL 19
BL 20
BL 21

M. latissimus
dorsi

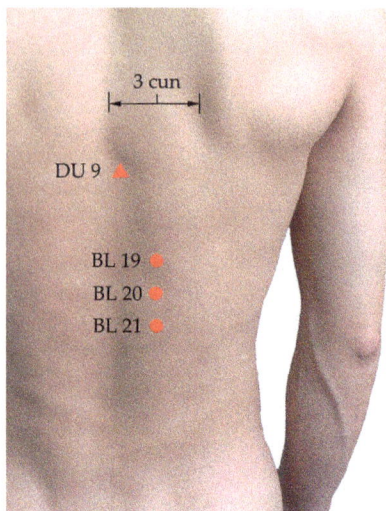

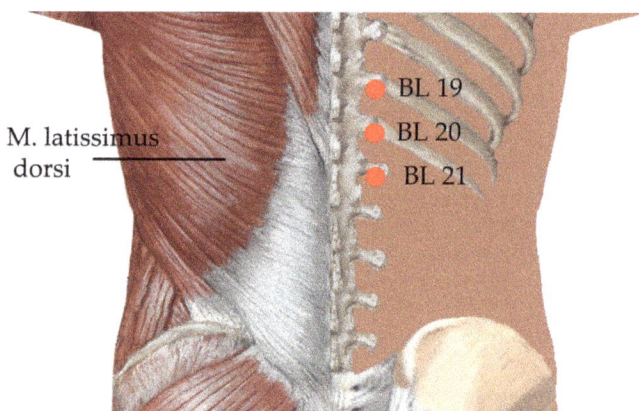

BL-22 Sānjiāoshū — Back-shu point of SJ

[Action]	Regulates sanjiao and regulates the fluid passage and promotes urination, benefits original Qi, tonifies the lumbar region and knees.
[Position]	On the lower back, 1.5 cun lateral to the lower border of the spinous process of the first lumbar vertebra.
[Acupuncture and Moxibustion]	**Acupuncture:** Insert the needle perpendicularly 0.8~1.0 cun deep. **Moxibustion:** Apply 5-9 moxa cones or needle-warming moxibustion or place a moxa stick above the point for 10~20 minutes.
[Indications]	Edema, dysuria and enuresis, borborygums, diarrhea and lumbago.

3 cun

DU 9

BL 22

M. latissimus dorsi

BL 22

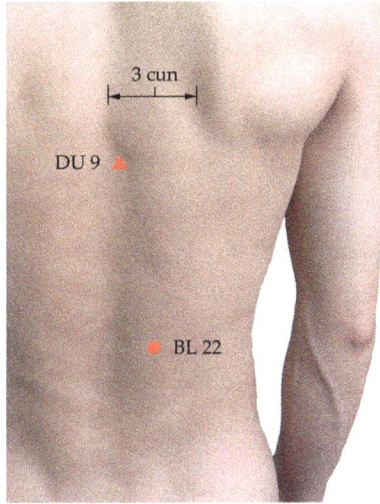

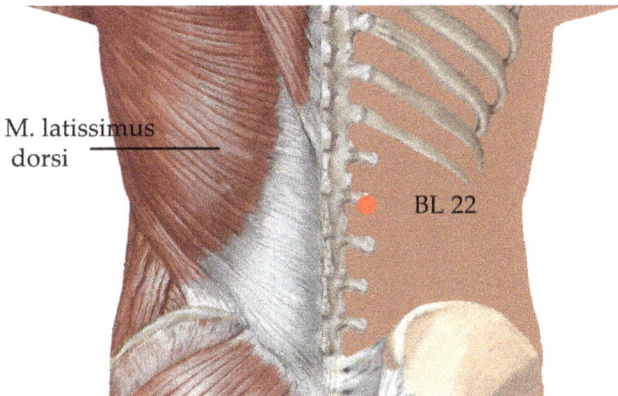

BL-23 Shènshū — Back-shu point of KI

[Action]	Strengthens kidney Qi and lumbar region, fortifies yang and regulates the fluid passage, benefits the ears and eyes.
[Position]	On the lower back, 1.5 cun lateral to the lower border of the spinous process of the second lumbar vertebra.
[Acupuncture and Moxibustion]	**Acupuncture:** Insert the needle perpendicularly 0.8~1.0 cun deep. **Moxibustion:** Apply 5-9 moxa cones or place a moxa stick above the point for 10~20 minutes.
[Indications]	Spermatorrhea, impotence, irregular menstruation, morbid leucorrhea, infertility, enuresis, adverse urination, edema, pain and soreness of the lower back and knees, blurred vision, tinnitus and deafness.

BL-25 Dàchángshū — Back-shu point of LI

[Action]	Regulates the intestines and stomach, regulates Qi and removes stagnation.
[Position]	On the lower back, 1.5 cun lateral to the lower border of the spinous process of the fourth lumbar vertebra.
[Acupuncture and Moxibustion]	**Acupuncture:** Insert the needle perpendicularly 0.8~1.0 cun deep. **Moxibustion:** Apply 5-9 moxa cones or place a moxa stick above the point for 10~20 minutes.
[Indications]	Abdominal pain and distention, diarrhea, borborygmus, constipation, dysentery and lumbago.

BL-27 Xiǎochángshū — Back-shu point of SI

[Action]	Clears heat and resolves dampness, regulates defecation.
[Position]	On the lower back, 1.5 cun lateral to the lower border of the spinous process of the first sacral vertebra.
[Acupuncture and Moxibustion]	**Acupuncture:** Insert the needle perpendicularly 0.8~1.0 cun deep **Moxibustion:** Apply 5-7 moxa cones or place a moxa stick above the point for 10~20 minutes.
[Indications]	Dysentery, diarrhea, hernia and hemorrhoids.

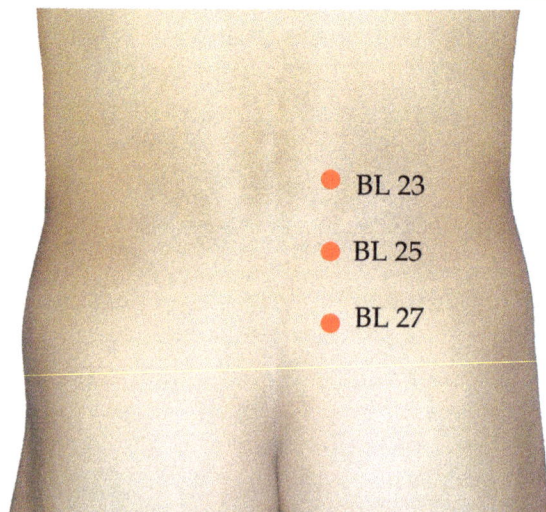

● BL 23

● BL 25

● BL 27

M. latissimus
dorsi

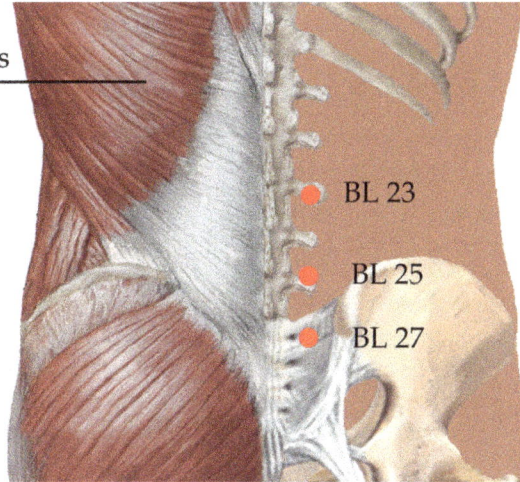

BL 23

BL 25

BL 27

BL-28 Pángguāngshū — Back-shu point of BL

[Action]	Clears heat and promotes diuresis, cultivates and re-plenishes the lower yuan.
[Position]	On the sacrum, 1.5 cun lateral to the middle of the sacral crest, at the level with the second posterior sacral foramen.
[Acupuncture and Moxibustion]	**Acupuncture:** Insert the needle perpendicularly 0.8-1.0 cun deep. **Moxibustion:** Apply 5-7 moxa cones or place a moxa stick above the point for 10~20 minutes.
[Indications]	Difficulty and redness of the urination, hesitancy and obstruction, enuresis and spermatorrhea.

BL 28

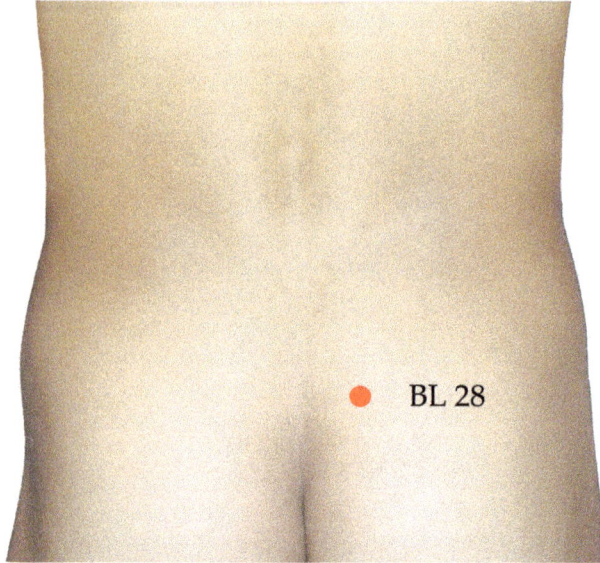

M. latissimus dorsi

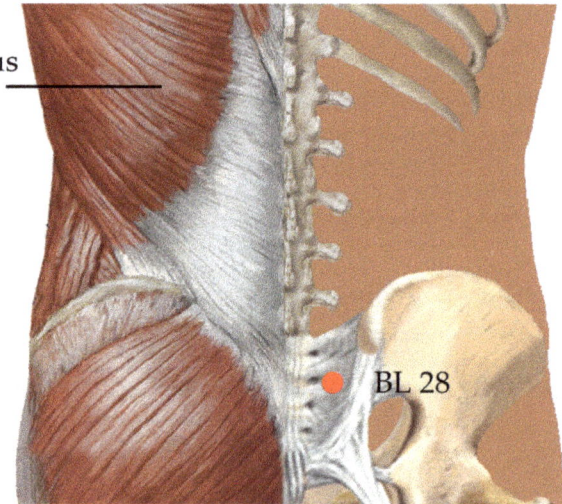

BL 28

CHAPTER 6

Front-mu Points

LU-1 Zhóngfǔ — Front-mu points of LU

[Action]	Alleviates cough and wheezing, clears lung and heat, tonifies Qi and invigorates the spleen.
[Position]	On the chest at the level with the first intercostals, 6 cun lateral to the front midline, in the depression lateral to the subclavian fossa.
[Acupuncture and Moxibustion]	**Acupuncture:** Insert the needle perpendicularly 0.3~0.5 cun deep and avoid deep insertion to prevent puncturing the anocelia. **Moxibustion:** Apply 3-5 moxa cones or place a moxa stick above the point for 10~20 minutes.
[Indications]	Cough, asthma, coughs and vomits purulent blood swelling and distention of the chest and the diaphragm.

CV-14 Jùquè — Front-mu points of HT

[Action]	Transforms phlegm and calms heart, regulates Qi and harmonizes stomach.
[Position]	On the upper abdomen, on the anterior midline, 6 cun superior to the umbilicus.
[Acupuncture and Moxibustion]	**Acupuncture:** Insert the needle perpendicularly 0.3~0.5 cun deep. **Moxibustion:** Apply 5-7 moxa cones or place a moxa stick above the point for 10~20 minutes or natural moxibustion.
[Indications]	Chest pain, cardiac pain, palpitations, epilepsy, nausea, vomiting and stomach ache.

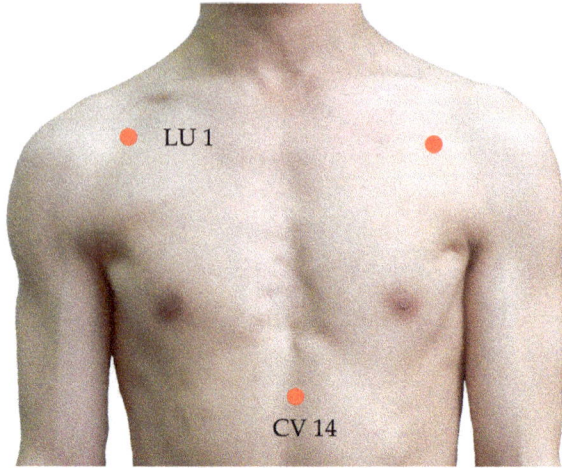

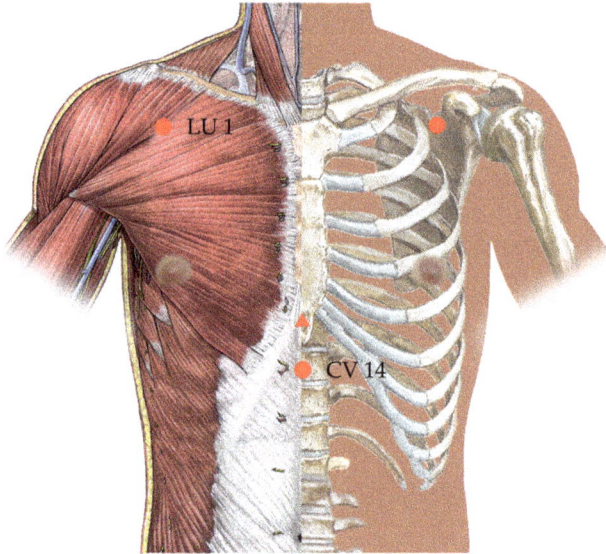

CV-17 Tánzhōng — Front-mu points of PC

[Action]	Unbinds the chest and regulates Qi, alleviates cough and wheezing.
[Position]	On the chest, on the anterior midline, at the level of the fourth intercostal space, at the midpoint between the two nipples.
[Acupuncture and Moxibustion]	**Acupuncture:** Insert the needle perpendicularly 0.3~0.5 cun deep. **Moxibustion:** Apply 5-9 moxa cones or place a moxa stick above the point for 10~20 minutes or natural moxibustion.
[Indications]	Chest distention, cough and asthma, choking diaphragm, insufficient lactation, infantile milk regurgitation.

LR-14 Qīmén — Front-mu points of LR

[Action]	Suppresses hyperactive liver and subsides yang, soothing liver-qi stagnation and invigorates spleen.
[Position]	On the chest, directly inferior to the nipple, in the sixth intercostal space, 4 cun lateral to the anterior midline.
[Acupuncture and Moxibustion]	**Acupuncture:** Insert the needle obliquely or subcutaneously along the intercostal space 0.5~0.8 cun deep. **Moxibustion:** Apply 5-9 moxa cones or place a moxa stick above the point for 10~20 minutes.
[Indications]	Distention of the chest and hypochondrium, pain of the hypochondrium, vomiting, hiccup and a lump in the abdomen.

LR-13 Zhāngmén — Front-mu points of SP

[Action]	Soothing liver-qi stagnation and invigorates spleen, descends rebellious Qi and relieves asthma.
[Position]	On the lateral aspect of the abdomen, below the free end of the eleventh floating rib.
[Acupuncture and Moxibustion]	Acupuncture: Insert the needle obliquely 0.5~0.8 cun, and avoid deep insertion to prevent puncturing the liver or spleen. Moxibustion: Apply 5-9 moxa cones or place a moxa stick above the point for 10~20 minutes.
[Indications]	Abdominal distention, diarrhea, vomiting, edema, distention of the chest and hypochondrium, jaundice and a lump in the abdomen.

GB-25 Jīngmén — Front-mu points of KI

[Action]	Induces diuresis and tonifies kidney and warms yang.
[Position]	On the lateral aspect of the upper abdomen, on the lower border of the end of the twelfth floating rib.
[Acupuncture and Moxibustion]	**Acupuncture:** Insert the needle obliquely 0.5~1.0 cun deep: **Moxibustion:** Apply 5-9 moxa cones or place a moxa stick above the point for 10~20 minutes.
[Indications]	Pain in the hypochondrium, abdominal distention and pain of the lumbar region.

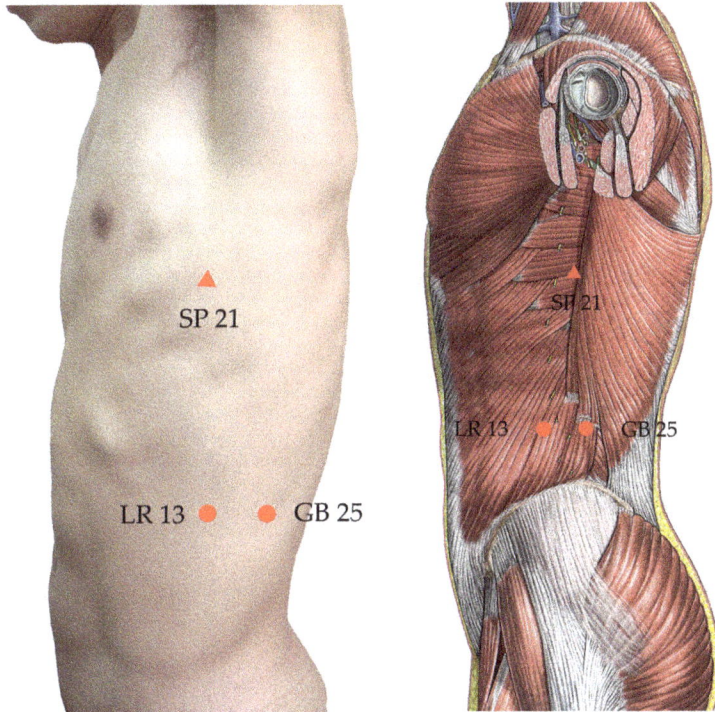

SP 21

LR 13 ● ● GB 25

CV-12 Zhōngwǎn — Front-mu points of ST

[Action]	Invigorates the spleen and harmonizes the stomach, warms middle jiao and removes dampness.
[Position]	On the upper abdomen, on the anterior midline, 4 cun superior to the umbilicus.
[Acupuncture and Moxibustion]	**Acupuncture:** Insert the needle perpendicularly 0.5~1.0 cun deep. **Moxibustion:** Apply 5-9 moxa cones or place a moxa stick above the point for 10~20 minutes. Scarring moxibustion can be used in health care, once a year, or indirect moxibustion 3-5 cones, or warm moxibustion to make local warm and red halo slightly, once a day, 20 times a month, this point can also use cumulative moxibustion.
[Indications]	Various diseases of the spleen and stomach: heatstroke, irritability, madness and epilepsy, syncope, headache, wheezing, irregular menstruation, amenorrhea, malignant obstruction of pregnancy.

GB-24 Rìyuè — Front-mu points of GB

[Action]	Lowers rebellious Qi and benefits the gall bladder, harmonizes intestine and stomach.
[Position]	On the chest, directly below the nipple in the seventh intercostal space, 4 cun lateral to the anterior midline.
[Acupuncture and Moxibustion]	**Acupuncture:** Insert the needle obliquely or subcutaneously along the intercostal space 0.5~0.8 cun deep. **Moxibustion:** Apply 3-5 moxa cones or place a moxa stick above the point for 10~20 minutes.
[Indications]	Hiccups, vomiting, stomach ache, abdominal distention and jaundice.

ST-25 Tiānshū — Front-mu points of LI

[Action]	Regulates the spleen and stomach, regulates Qi and invigorates the spleen.
[Position]	On the abdomen, 2 cun lateral to the umbilicus.
[Acupuncture and Moxibustion]	**Acupuncture:** Insert the needle perpendicularly 1.0~1.5 cun deep: **Moxibustion:** Apply 5-10 moxa cones or place a moxa stick above the point for 15~30 minutes.
[Indications]	Vomiting, hematemesis, borborygmus, abdominal distention, pain around the umbilicus, dysentery, constipation and hernia.

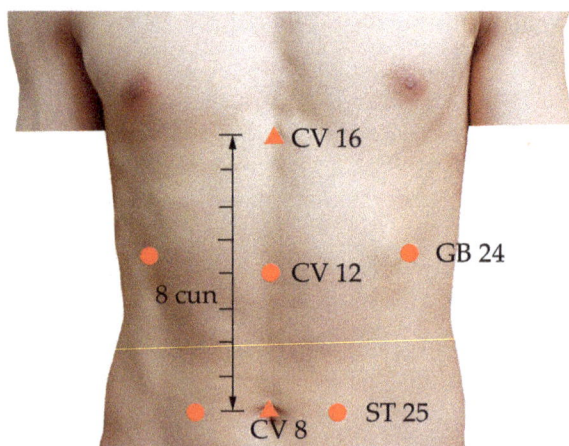

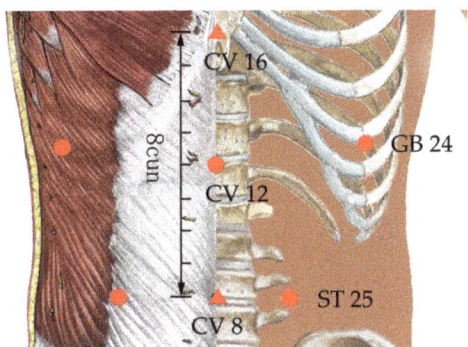

CV 16
8cun
CV 12
GB 24
ST 25
CV 8

CV-3 Zhōngjí — Front-mu points of BL

[Action]	Transforms dampness (the state of body feeling damp) and clears heat, benefits kidney and regulates menstruation, activates yang and transforms Qi.
[Position]	On the lower abdomen, on the anterior midline, 4 cun inferior to the umbilicus.
[Acupuncture and Moxibustion]	**Acupuncture:** Insert the needle perpendicularly 0.5~1.0 cun deep and stimulate until there is a sore and distending sensation in the local area radiating to the genitalia. Request for the patient to empty their bladder before the puncturing this point, avoid puncturing the bladder and the intestines. Acupuncture and moxibustion is prohibited during pregnancy. **Moxibustion:** Apply 5-7 moxa cones or place a moxa stick above the point for 10~20 minutes.
[Indications]	Herina, spermatorrhea, enuresis, difficulty in urination, pruritus and pain of vulvae, irregular menstruation.

CV-5 Shímén — Front-mu points of TE

[Action]	Invigorates spleen and tonifies kidney and regulates sanjiao.
[Position]	On the lower abdomen, on the anterior midline, 2 cun inferior to the umbilicus.
[Acupuncture and Moxibustion]	**Acupuncture:** Insert the needle perpendicularly 0.5~1.0 cun deep. **Moxibustion:** Apply 5-9 moxa cones or place a moxa stick above the point for 10~20 minutes.
[Indications]	Amenorrhea and morbid leucorrhea, edema and difficulty in urination.

CV-4 Guānyuán — Front-mu points of SI

[Action]	Tonifies yuan to stop collapse, warms kidney and strengthens yang, regulates menstruation and leucorrhea.
[Position]	On the lower abdomen, on the anterior midline, 3 cun inferior to the umbilicus.
[Acupuncture and Moxibustion]	**Acupuncture:** Insert the needle perpendicularly 0.5~1.0 cun deep. **Moxibustion:** Apply 5-9 moxa cones or place a moxa stick above the point for 10~20 minutes. Scarring moxibustion can be used in health care, once a year, or indirect moxibustion or warm moxibustion to make local warm and comfort with red ring, once a day, 20 times a month, this point can also use cumulative moxibustion more than 100 cones.
[Indications]	Diseases of the lower abdomen, gynecological disorders, disorders of the stomach and intestines, weakness.

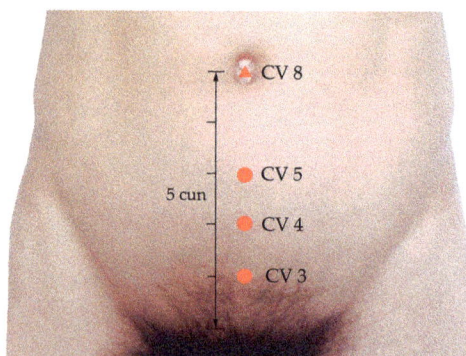

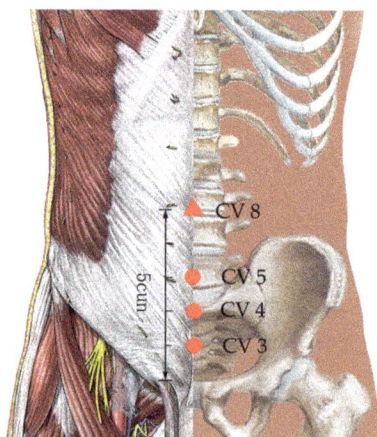

CHAPTER 7

Eight Confluence Points

SI-3 Hòuxī — Confluent points of the Du vessel:
Shu-stream point of SI

[Action]	Clears the head and brightens the eyes, calms the spirit and treats epilepsy, dredges the channel and actives the collatrals.
[Position]	On the ulnar side of the hand, proximal to the fifth metacarpophalangeal joint, at the end of the transverse crease, at the junction of the red and white skin side.
[Acupuncture and Moxibustion]	**Acupuncture:** Insert the needle perpendicularly 0.5~0.8 cun deep. **Moxibustion:** Apply 1-3 moxa cones or place a moxa stick above the point for 5~10 minutes.
[Indications]	Febrile diseases with anhidrosis, jaundice, malaria, painful eyes and lacrimation, superficial visual obstruction, swelling of cheeks, swollen and sore throat, psychosis, epilepsy, hysteria, insomnia, stroke, pain and rigidity of the head and neck, spasmodic pain and numbness of the elbow, arm and little finger, paralysis.

TE-5 Wàiguān — Confluent points of the yang linking vessel: Luo-connecting point of TE

[Action]	Clears heat and releases exterior, dredges the channel and activates the collaterals.
[Position]	On the dorsal side of the forearm, 2 cun proximal to the transverse crease of the wrist, in the depression between the ulna and radius.
[Acupuncture and Moxibustion]	**Acupuncture:** Insert the needle perpendicularly or obliquely 0.5~1.0 cun deep. **Moxibustion:** Apply 3-5 moxa cones or needle-warming moxibustion or place a moxa stick above the point for 10~20 minutes.
[Indications]	Febrile diseases, common cold, headache, tinnitus, chest and hypochondriac pain, inability to raise arm.

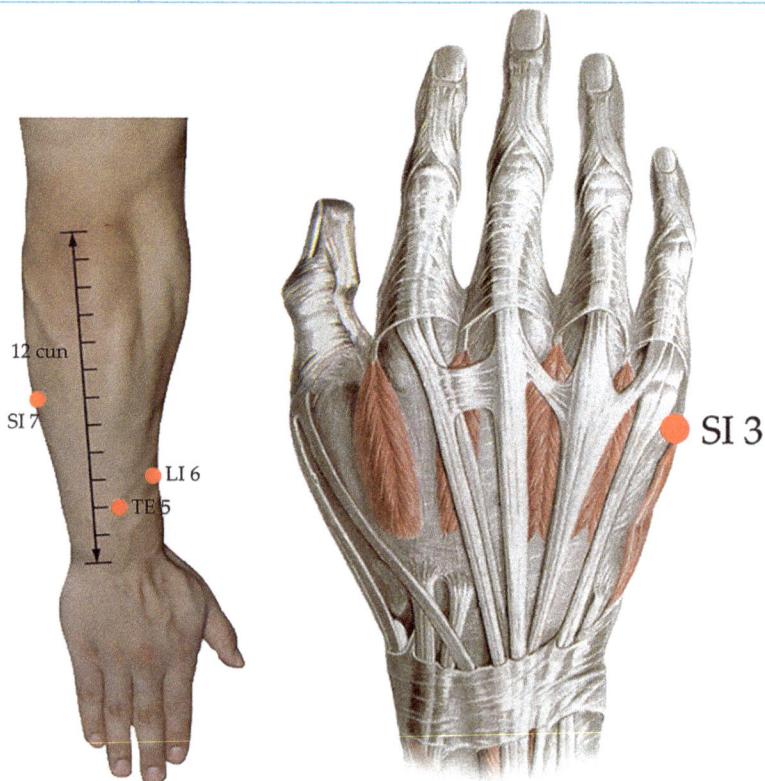

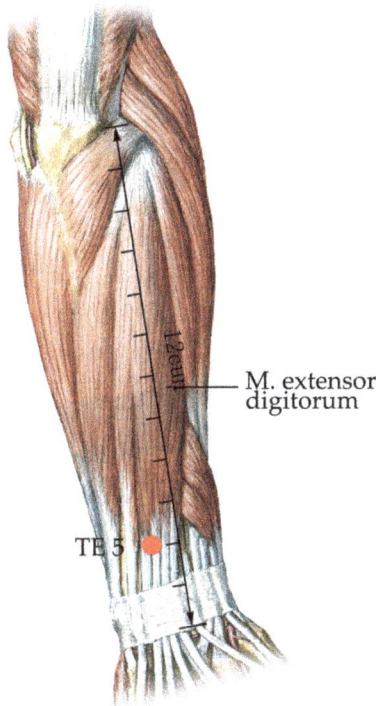

M. extensor
digitorum

TE 5

LU-7 Lièquē — Confluent points of the Du vessel: Luo-connecting point of LU

[Action]	Releases the exterior and expels wind, regulates the Ren vessel.
[Position]	On the radial side of the forearm, 1.5 cun proximal the transverse crease of the wrist, superior to the styolid process of the radius and between tendons of m. brachioradialis and m. abductor pollicis longus.
[Acupuncture and Moxibustion]	**Acupuncture:** Insert the needle obliquely upward 0.2~0.3 cun deep. **Moxibustion:** Apply 3-5 moxa cones or place a moxa stick above the point for 5~10 minutes.
[Indications]	Cough, asthma, shortness of breath, headache and migraine, neck stiffness and sore throat,

PC-6 Nèiguān — Confluent point of the yin linking vessel: Luo-connecting point of PC

[Action]	Regulates heart and calms the spirit, descends rebellious Qi and regulates stomach, unbinds the chest and regulates Qi, clears heat and alleviates pain.
[Position]	On the palmar aspect of the forearm, 2 cun superior to the transverse crease of the wrist, between the tendon of palmaris longus and flexor carpi radialis.
[Acupuncture and Moxibustion]	**Acupuncture:** Insert the needle perpendicularly 0.5~1.5 cun deep. **Moxibustion:** Apply 5-7 moxa cones or place a moxa stick above the point for 10~20 minutes.
[Indications]	Cardiac pain, palpitation, insomnia, stomach ache, vomiting, hiccough and asthma.

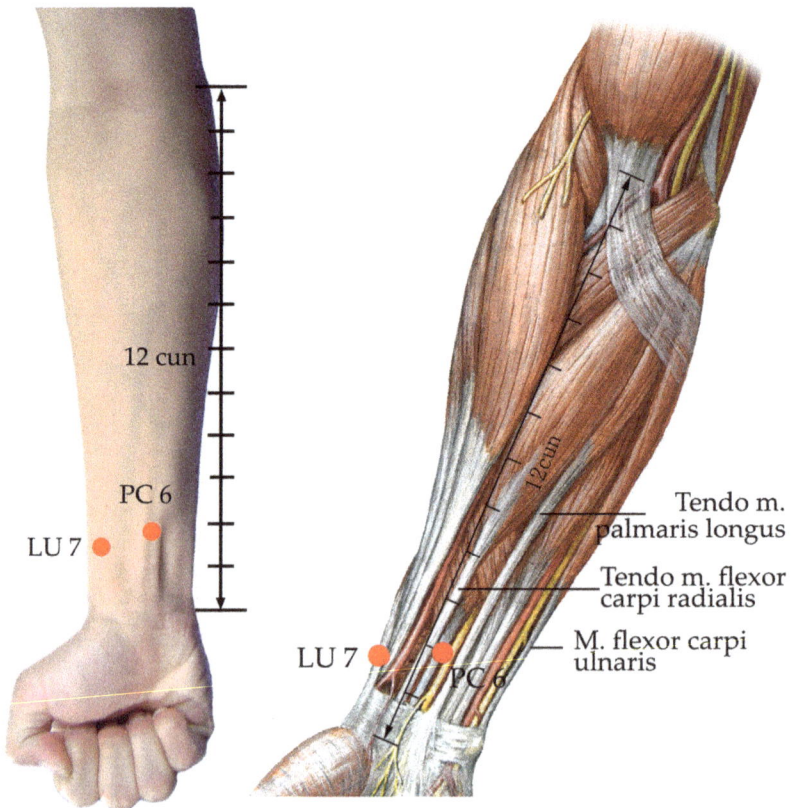

12 cun

PC 6

LU 7

12 cun

Tendo m. palmaris longus

Tendo m. flexor carpi radialis

LU 7   PC 6

M. flexor carpi ulnaris

SP-4 Gōngsūn — Confluent point of the Chong vessel: Luo-connecting point of SP

[Action]	Invigorates the spleen and stomach, regulates the Chong vessels and Ren vessels.
[Position]	On the medial side of the foot, in the depression anterior and inferior to the base of the first metatarsal bone, at the junction of the red and white skin.
[Acupuncture and Moxibustion]	**Acupuncture:** Insert the needle perpendicularly 0.5~0.8 cun deep. **Moxibustion:** Apply 3-5 moxa cones or place a moxa stick above the point for 10-20 minutes.
[Indications]	Vomiting, abdominal pain, stomach ache, borborygums, diarrhea and dysentery.

KI-6 Zhàohǎi — Confluent points of the yin motility vessel

[Action]	Nourishes yin and regulates menstruation, pacifies wind and removes spasm, relieves sore-throat and calms spirit.
[Position]	On the medial side of the foot, 1 cun inferior to the tip of the medial malleous, in the depression inferior to the tip of the medial malleous.
[Acupuncture and Moxibustion]	**Acupuncture:** Insert the needle perpendicularly or obliquely upward 0.5~0.8 cun deep. **Moxibustion:** Apply 3-5 moxa cones or place a moxa stick above the point for 5~10 minutes.
[Indications]	Swelling and pain of the throat, sudden loss of voice, heartache, asthma, constipation, diarrhea, irregular menstruation, dysmenorrhea, amenorrhea, woman's anemic fainting, retention of afterbirth, persistent lochia, hernia, gonorrhea, spermatorrhea, urinary retention, frequent urination, enuresis, epilepsy and panic.

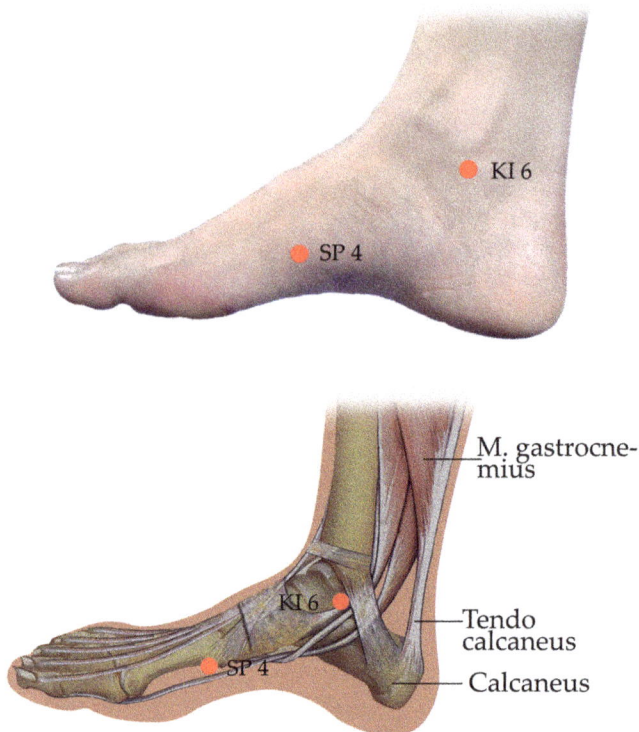

KI 6

SP 4

M. gastrocnemius

KI 6

SP 4

Tendo calcaneus

Calcaneus

GB-41 Zúlínqì — Confluent point of the girdling vessel: Shu-stream point of GB

[Action]	Soothing liver-qi stagnation and resolves depression, pacifies wind and clears fire.
[Position]	On the lateral aspect of the dorsum of the foot, distal to the junction of the 4th and 5th metatarsal bone, in the depression on the lateral aspect of the tendon of m. extensor digit minimi of the foot.
[Acupuncture and Moxibustion]	**Acupuncture:** Insert the needle perpendicularly 0.5~0.8 cun deep. **Moxibustion:** Apply 3-5moxa cones or place a moxa stick above the point for 5~10 minutes.
[Indications]	Headache and dizziness, redness, swelling and pain of the eye, toothache, swollen throat, deafness, mastitis, dyspnea, swelling and pain in the axillary region, pain in the hypochondrium, pain of the knee and ankle and redness and swelling of the dorsum of the foot.

BL-62 Shēnmài — Confluent points of the yang motility vessel

[Action]	Activates blood and regulates Qi, calms spirit and heart.
[Position]	On the lateral side of the foot, in the depression inferior to the tip of external malleolus, between the inferior margin of the external malleolus and calcaneus.
[Acupuncture and Moxibustion]	**Acupuncture:** Insert the needle perpendicularly or obliquely upward 0.2~0.3 cun deep. **Moxibustion:** Apply 3-5 moxa cones or place a moxa stick above the point for 5~10 minutes.
[Indications]	Insomnia, manic psychosis, epilepsy, headache, stroke and unconsciousness, migraine and vertigo.

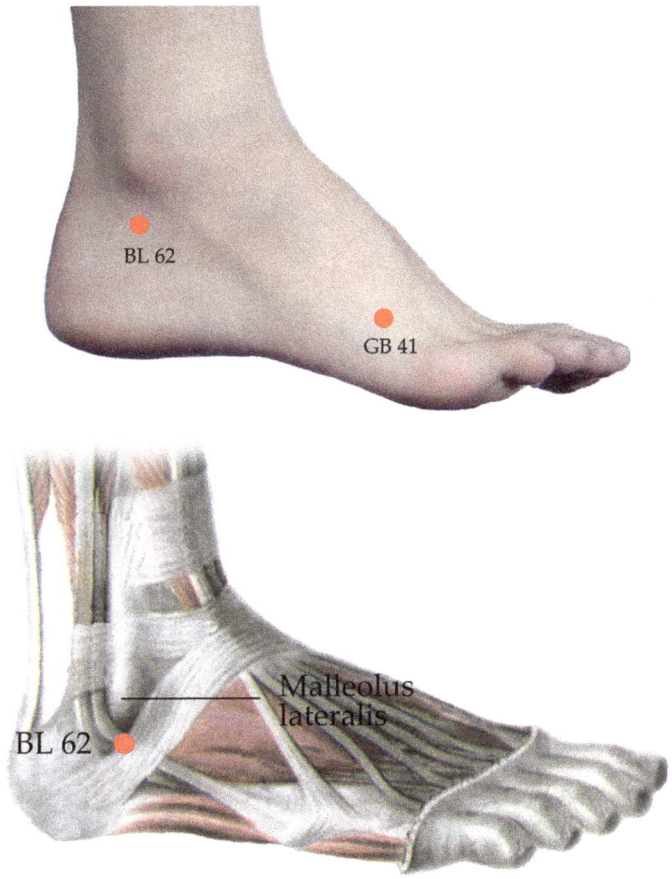

BL 62

GB 41

Malleolus lateralis

BL 62

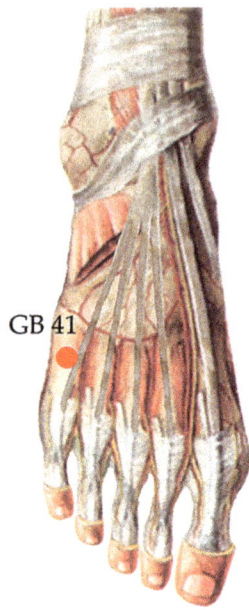

GB 41

CHAPTER 8

Eight Influential Points

CV-12 Zhōngwǎn — Influential point of the Fu: Front-mu points of ST

[Action]	Invigorates spleen and harmonizes stomach, warms middle jiao and removes dampness.
[Position]	On the upper abdomen, on the anterior midline, 4 cun superior to the umbilicus.
[Acupuncture and Moxibustion]	**Acupuncture:** Insert the needle perpendicularly 0.5~1.0 cun deep: **Moxibustion:** Apply 5-9 moxa cones or place a moxa stick above the point for 10~20 minutes. Scarring moxibustion can be used in health care, once a year, or indirect moxibustion 3-5 cones, or warm moxibustion to make location warm with a slight red ring, once a day, 20 times a month, this point can also use cumulative moxibustion.
[Indications]	Various diseases of spleen and stomach: heatstroke, irritability, madness and epilepsy, syncope, headache, wheezing, irregular menstruation, amenorrhea, malignant obstruction of pregnancy.

LR-13 Zhāngmén — Influential point of the Zang: Front-mu points of SP

[Action]	Soothing liver-qi stagnation and invigorates spleen, descends rebellious Qi and relieves asthma.
[Position]	On the lateral aspect of the abdomen, below the free end of the eleventh floating rib.
[Acupuncture and Moxibustion]	**Acupuncture:** Insert the needle obliquely 0.5~0.8 cun, and avoid deep insertion to prevent puncturing the liver or spleen. **Moxibustion:** Apply 5-9 moxa cones or place a moxa stick above the point for 10~20 minutes.
[Indications]	Abdominal distention, diarrhea, vomiting, edema, distention of the chest and hypochondrium, jaundice and a lump in the abdomen

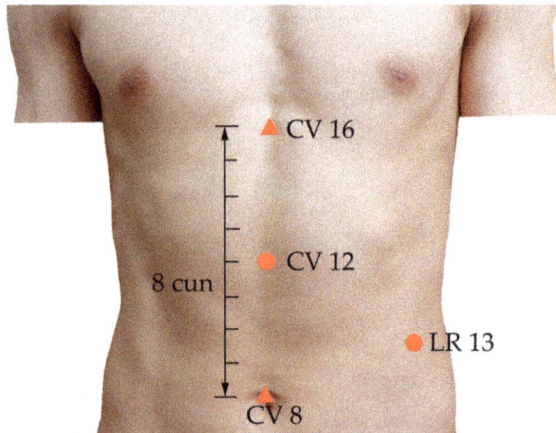

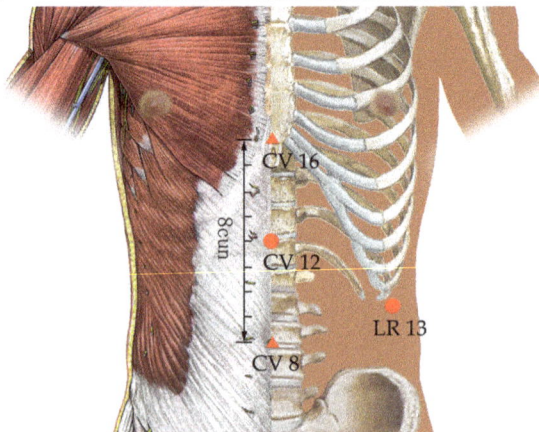

CV-17 Tánzhōng — Influential point of Qi: Front-mu points of PC

[Action]	Unbinds the chest and regulates Qi, alleviates cough and wheezing.
[Position]	On the chest, on the anterior midline, at the level of the fourth intercostal space, at the midpoint between the two nipples.
[Acupuncture and Moxibustion]	**Acupuncture:** Insert the needle perpendicularly 0.3~0.5 cun deep. **Moxibustion:** Apply 5-9 moxa cones or place a moxa stick above the point for 10~20 minutes or natural moxibustion.
[Indications]	Chest distention, cough and asthma, chocking diaphragm, Insufficient lactation, infantile milk regurgitation.

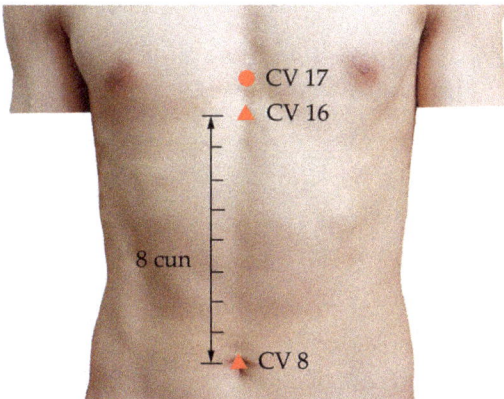

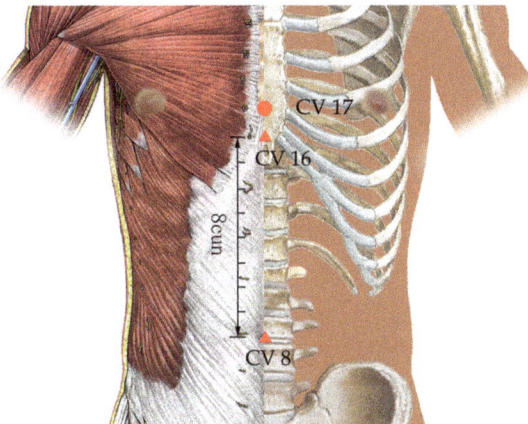

BL-11 Dàzhù — Influential point of the bone

[Action]	Expels wind and clears heat tonifies the bones and sinews.
[Position]	On the upper back, 1.5 cun lateral to the lower border of the spinous process of the first thoracic vertebra.
[Acupuncture and Moxibustion]	**Acupuncture:** Insert the needle obliquely towards the spine 0.5~0.8 cun deep. **Moxibustion:** Apply 5-7 moxa cones or place a moxa stick above the point for 10-20 minutes.
[Indications]	Neck stiffness, pain in the shoulder and back, asthma and distention of the chest and hypochondrium.

BL-17 Géshū — Influential point of the blood.

[Action]	Regulates and descends rebellious Qi, activates blood circulation and dredges the collaterals.
[Position]	On the back, 1.5 cun lateral to the lower border of the spinous process of the seventh thoracic vertebra.
[Acupuncture and Moxibustion]	**Acupuncture:** Insert the needle obliquely towards the spine 0.5~0.8 cun deep. **Moxibustion:** Apply 5-7 moxa cones or place a moxa stick above the point for 10-20 minutes.
[Indications]	Blood syndrome such as hemoptysis, bleeding, blood in the stools, postpartum bleeding, cardiac pain, palpitation, chest pain, chest distend, vomiting, hiccup, night sweating, urticaria.

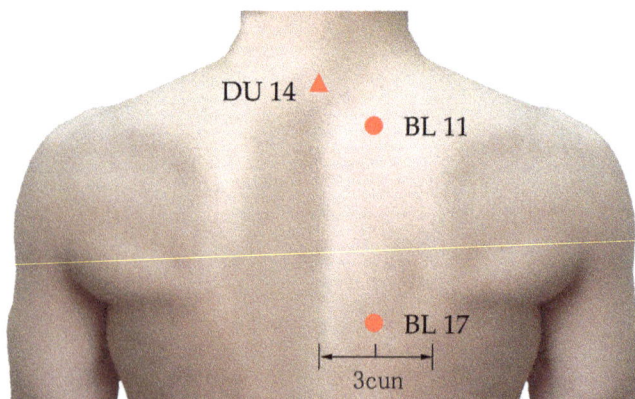

DU 14
BL 11
BL 17
3cun

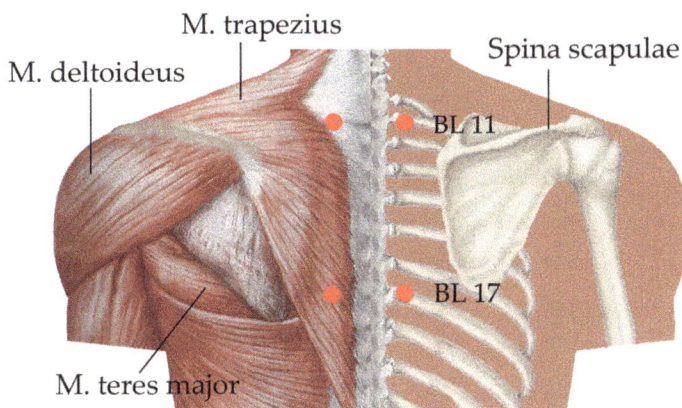

M. trapezius

M. deltoideus

Spina scapulae

BL 11

BL 17

M. teres major

LU-9 Tàiyuān — Shu-stream point of LU: Influential point of the vessels

[Action]	Alleviates cough and transforms phlegm, regulates and harmonizes the vessels, tonifies Qi and invigorates the spleen
[Position]	On the radial end of the wrist crease, in depression ulnar to the m. abductor pollicis longus, between the styloid process of radius and scaphoid bone
[Acupuncture and Moxibustion]	**Acupuncture:** Insert the needle perpendicularly 0.2~0.3 cun deep. Avoid puncturing the radial artery. **Moxibustion:** Apply 1-3 moxa cones or place a moxa stick above the point for 5-10 minutes.
[Indications]	Cough, asthma, chest congestion, palpitations and pulseless disease.

GB-34 Yánglíngquán Influential point of the sinews: Lower he-sea point of GB: He-sea point of GB

[Action]	Clears heat and pacifies wind, relieves swelling and alleviates pain.
[Position]	On the lateral aspect of the lower leg, in the depression anterior and inferior to the head of the fibula.
[Acupuncture and Moxibustion]	**Acupuncture:** Insert the needle perpendicularly towards SP9 (Yīnlíngquán) 1.0~3.0 cun deep **Moxibustion:** Apply 3-5 moxa cones or place a moxa stick above the point for 5~10minutes.
[Indications]	Headache, tinnitus, deafness, eye pain, swollen cheeks, pain of the chest and hypochondrium, swelling and pain of the breast, asthma, cough, chest distention, vomiting, jaundice, swelling and pain of the knee, weakness and numbness of the lower extremities, spasm, softness, contraction and tightness of the sinews, beriberi and hemiplegia

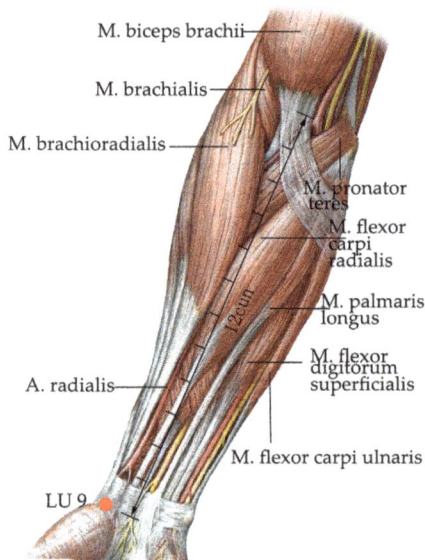

M. biceps brachii

M. brachialis

M. brachioradialis

M. pronator teres

M. flexor carpi radialis

12cun

M. palmaris longus

M. flexor digitorum superficialis

A. radialis

M. flexor carpi ulnaris

LU 9

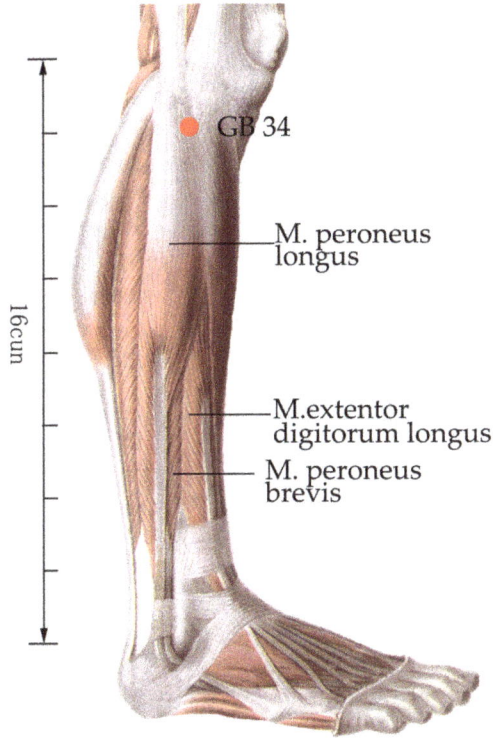

GB 34

M. peroneus longus

M.extentor digitorum longus

M. peroneus brevis

16cun

GB-39 Xuánzhōng — Influential point of the marrow

[Action]	Benefits marrow and produces blood, relaxes sinews and activates the collaterals.
[Position]	On the lateral aspect of the lower leg, 3 cun proximal to the tip of the external malleolus, anterior border of fibula.
[Acupuncture and Moxibustion]	**Acupuncture:** Insert the needle perpendicularly 1.0~2.0 cun deep. **Moxibustion:** Apply 3-5 moxa cones or needle-warming moxibustion or place a moxa stick above the point for 10-20 minutes.
[Indications]	Neck stiffness, pain of the chest and hypochondrium, swelling and pain in the axillary region, hemiplegia and pain of the heel, abdominal distention, dizziness, tinnitus and deafness, high blood pressure.

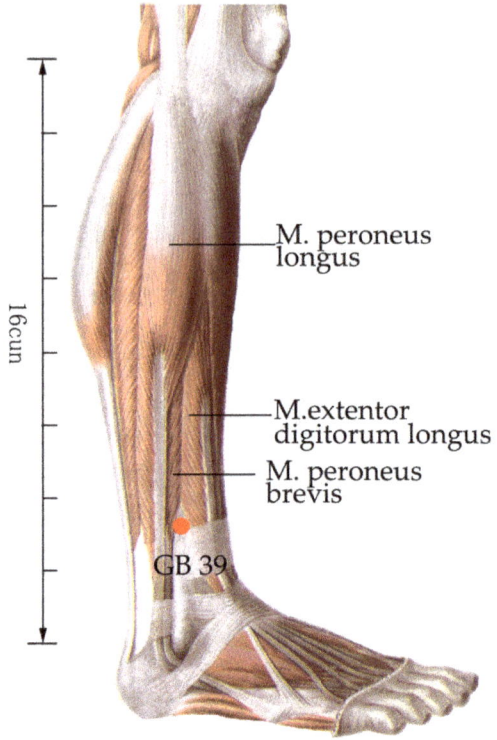

16cun

M. peroneus
longus

M.extentor
digitorum longus

M. peroneus
brevis

GB 39

CHAPTER 9

Xi-cleft Points

LI-7 Wēnliū — Xi-cleft point of LI

[Action]	Regulates and harmonizes the intestines and stomach, clears heat.
[Position]	On the radial side of the arm, 5 cun proximal to the crease the wrist on the line connecting LI 5 (Yángxī) and LI 11 (Qǔchí), when the elbow is flexed.
[Acupuncture and Moxibustion]	**Acupuncture:** Insert the needle perpendicularly 0.5~1.0 cun deep. Tenderness occurs at this point when perforation of digestive tract ulcer. **Moxibustion:** Apply 5-9 moxa cones or place a moxa stick above the point for 10~20 minutes.
[Indications]	Headache, redness and swelling of the face, pain of the mouth and tough, the ulcer of stomach and duodenum.

SI-6 Yǎnglǎo — Xi-cleft point of SI

[Action]	Brightens the eyes and clears heat, relaxes sinews and activates the collateral.
[Position]	On the ulnar rear of forearm, in the depression on the radial side of the styloid process of the ulna.
[Acupuncture and Moxibustion]	**Acupuncture:** Insert the needle obliquely upward 0.5~0.8 cun deep. **Moxibustion:** Apply 3-5 moxa cones or place a moxa stick above the point for 10~20 minutes.
[Indications]	Blurred vision, acute lumbago, headache and pain of the shoulder and back.

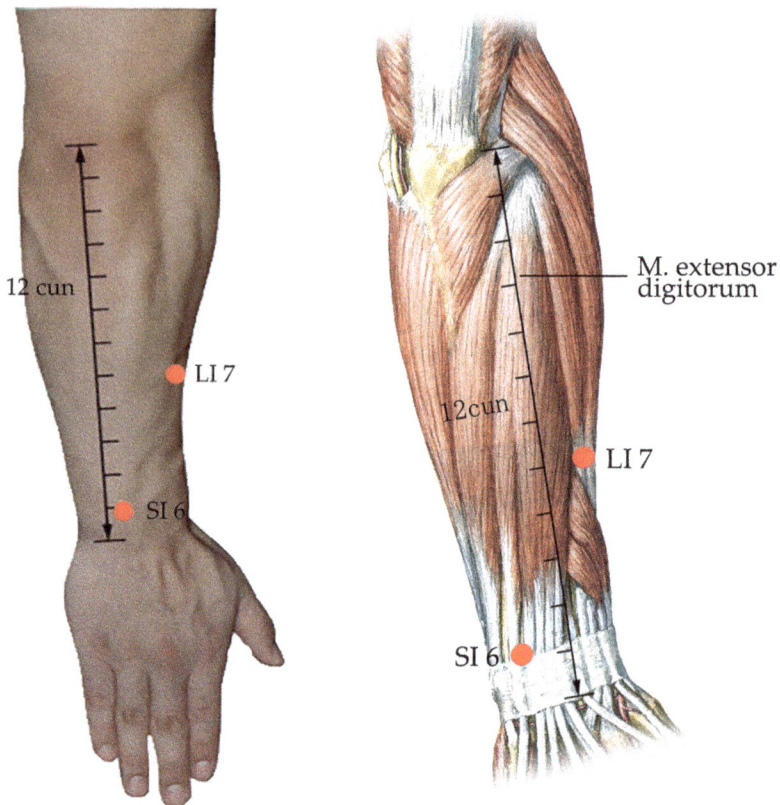

12 cun

LI 7

SI 6

M. extensor
digitorum

12cun

LI 7

SI 6

TE-7 Huìzōng — Xi-cleft point of TE

[Action]	Clears heat and calms the spirit, benefits ears and dredges the collaterals.
[Position]	On the dorsal side of the forearm, 3 cun proximal to the transverse wrist crease, on radial side of the ulna.
[Acupuncture and Moxibustion]	**Acupuncture:** Insert the needle obliquely upward 0.5~1.0 cun deep. **Moxibustion:** Apply 3-5 moxa cones or place a moxa stick above the point for 5~10 minutes.
[Indications]	Migraine, deafness and tinnitus, cough and asthma, chest distention and pain of the arm.

12cun

TE 7

M. extensor digitorum

12cun

TE 7

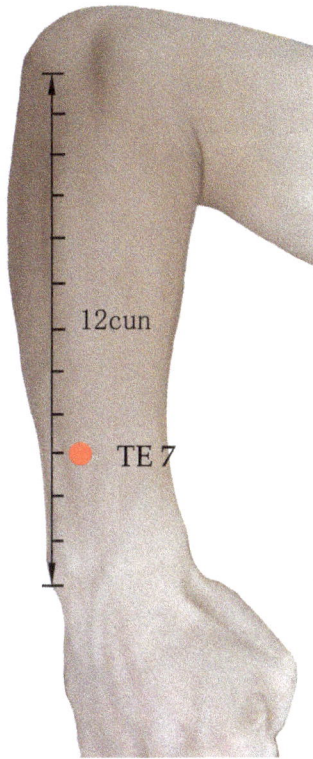

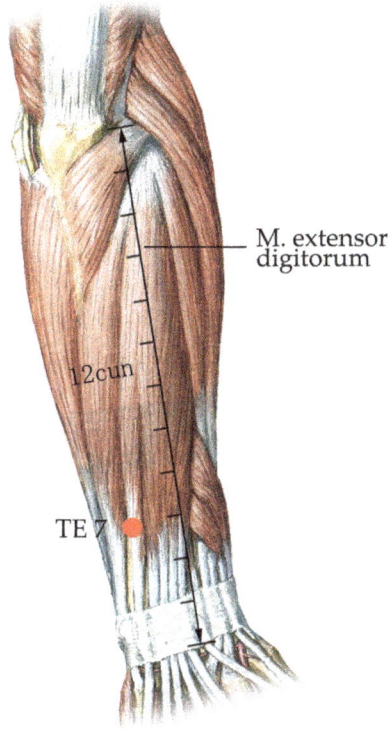

LU-6 Kǒngzuì — Xi-cleft point of LU

[Action]	Clears heat and removes toxins, disperses and descends lung qi and stops bleeding.
[Position]	On the line connecting LU 9 (Taiyuan) and LU 5 (Chize), 7 cun above the transverse crease of the wrist on the palmar aspect of the forearm.
[Acupuncture and Moxibustion]	**Acupuncture:** Insert the needle perpendicularly 0.5~0.8 cun deep. **Moxibustion:** apply 5-7 moxa cones or needle-warming moxibustion or place a moxa stick above the point for 10-20 minutes.
[Indications]	Hemoptysis, epistaxis, sore throat and pain of the arm.

PC-4 Xìmén — Xi-cleft point of PC

[Action]	Regulates Qi and alleviates pain, cools blood and stops bleeding, calms the spirit and heart.
[Position]	On the palmar side of the forearm, 5 cun superior to the transverse crease of the wrist, on the line connecting PC 3 (qū zé) to PC 7 (dà ling).
[Acupuncture and Moxibustion]	**Acupuncture:** Insert the needle perpendicularly 0.5~0.8 cun deep. **Moxibustion:** apply 3-5 moxa cones or needle-warming moxibustion or place a moxa stick above the point for 10-20 minutes.
[Indications]	Cardiac pain and palpitation, stomach ache and hemoptysis.

HT-6 Yīnxì — Xi-cleft point of HT

[Action]	Clears heat and calms the spirit, strengthen exterior and recovers voice.
[Position]	On the palmar side of the forearm, on the radial side of the tendon m. flexor carpi ulnaris, 0.5 cun proximal to the transverse wrist crease.
[Acupuncture and Moxibustion]	**Acupuncture:** Insert the needle perpendicularly 0.3~0.5 cun deep. **Moxibustion:** Apply 3 moxa cones or place a moxa stick above the point for 10-20 minutes.
[Indications]	Cardiac pain, cardiopalmus, night sweat and loss voice.

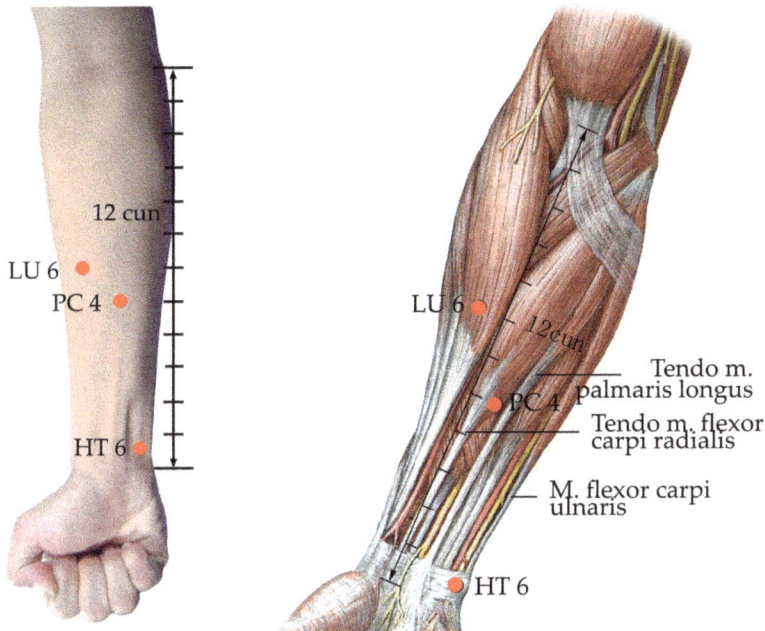

12 cun

LU 6

PC 4

HT 6

LU 6

12 cun

PC 4

Tendo m. palmaris longus

Tendo m. flexor carpi radialis

M. flexor carpi ulnaris

HT 6

KI-5 Shuǐquán — Xi-cleft point of KI

[Action]	Induces diuresis for removing edema, activates blood and regulates menstruation.
[Position]	On the medial side of the foot, posterior and inferior to the media malleolus l, 1 cun directly inferior to KI 3 (Tàixī), in the depression anterior to the tuberosity of the calcaneum.
[Acupuncture and Moxibustion]	**Acupuncture:** Insert the needle perpendicularly 0.3~0.5 cun deep: **Moxibustion:** Apply 3-5 moxa cones or place a moxa stick above the point for 5~10 minutes.
[Indications]	Difficulty in urination and pain of the heel.

LR-6 Zhōngdū — Xi-cleft point of LR

[Action]	Soothing liver-qi stagnation and regulates Qi, regulates menstruation and stops bleeding.
[Position]	On the medial aspect of the lower leg, 7 cun proximal to the tip of the medial malleolus, in the center of the medial aspect of the tibia.

[Acupuncture and Moxibustion]	**Acupuncture:** Insert the needle subcutaneously 0.5~0.8 cun deep. **Moxibustion:** apply 3-5 moxa cones or needle-warming moxibustion or place a moxa stick above the point for 5-10 minutes.
[Indications]	Hernia, spermatorrhea, metrorrhagia and retention of lochia.

SP-8 Dìjī — Xi-cleft point of SP

[Action]	Harmonizes the spleen and resolves dampness, regulates menstruation and arrests leucorrhoea.
[Position]	On the medial aspect of the lower leg, 3 cun inferior to SP 9 (Yīnlíngquán), posterior to the medial edge of the tibia.
[Acupuncture and Moxibustion]	**Acupuncture:** Insert the needle perpendicularly 1.0~1.5 cun deep. **Moxibustion:** Apply 3-5 moxa cones or place a moxa stick above the point for 5~10 minutes.
[Indications]	Abdominal distention and pain, anorexia, irregular menstruation.

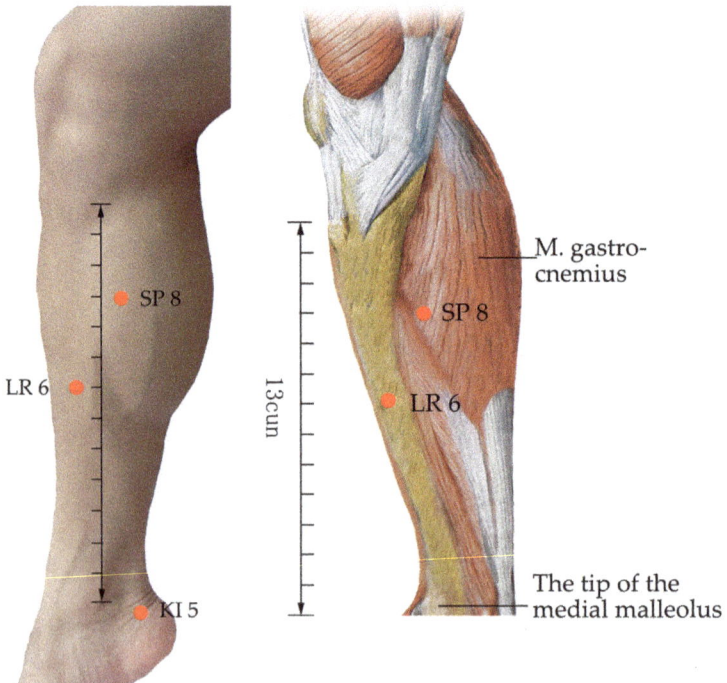

SP 8
LR 6
13cun
KI 5
M. gastro-cnemius
The tip of the medial malleolus

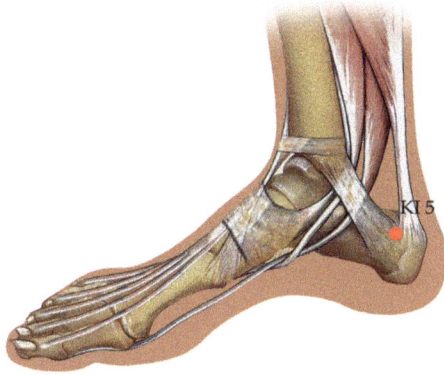

ST-34 Liángqiū — Xi-cleft point of ST

[Action]	Harmonizes the stomach and regulates Qi, dredges the channel and the collaterals.
[Position]	On the anterior aspect of the thigh, 2 cun proximal to the patella when the knee is bent, between the m. vastus lateralis and the tendons of the rectus femoris.
[Acupuncture and Moxibustion]	**Acupuncture:** Insert the needle perpendicularly 1.0~1.5 cun deep. **Moxibustion:** apply 7-9 moxa cones or needle-warming moxibustion or place a moxa stick above the point for 10-20 minutes.
[Indications]	Stomach ache, borborygmus and diarrhea, pain of the knee, leg and lumbago.

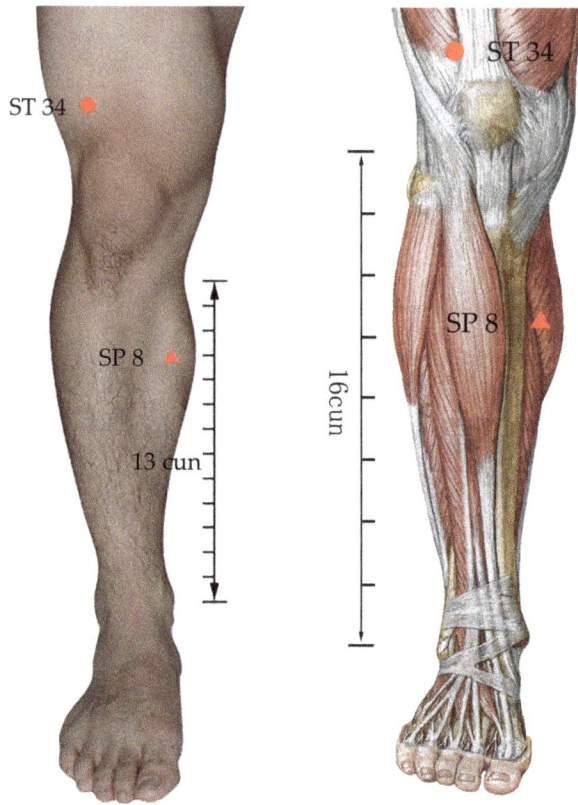

BL-63 Jīnmén — Xi-cleft point of BL

[Action]	Dredges the channel and activates the collaterals, clears head and calms spirit.
[Position]	On the lateral side of the foot, inferior to the anterior border of the external malleolus, lateral to the lower border of the cuboid bone.
[Acupuncture and Moxibustion]	**Acupuncture:** Insert the needle perpendicularly 0.3~0.5 cun deep. **Moxibustion:** Apply 3-5 moxa cones or place a moxa stick above the point for 5~10 minutes.
[Indications]	Intermittent headache, epilepsy, pain of the lower back and legs and foot sprain.

GB-36 Wàiqiū — Xi-cleft point of GB

[Action]	Soothing liver-qi stagnation and regulates Qi, dredges the channel and activates the collaterals.
[Position]	On the lateral aspect of the lower limb, 7 cun proximal to the tip of the external malleolus, on the anterior border of the fibula.
[Acupuncture and Moxibustion]	**Acupuncture:** Insert the needle perpendicularly 0.5~0.8 cun deep. **Moxibustion:** apply 3-5 moxa cones or needle-warming moxibustion or place a moxa stick above the point for 5-10 minutes.
[Indications]	Psychosis and vomiting, pain of the chest and the hypochondrium.

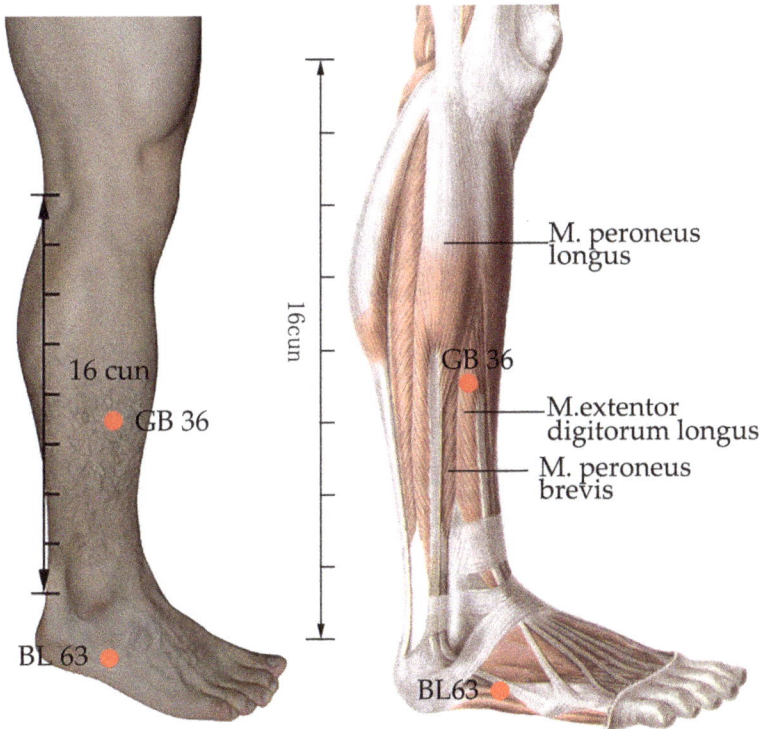

BL-59 Fūyáng — Xi-cleft point of the yang motility vessel

[Action]	Dredges the channel and activates, expels wind and clears heat.
[Position]	On the posterior aspect of the lower leg, posterior to the external mallelous, 3 cun superior to BL 60 (Kūn-lún), between the fibula and the heel tendon.
[Acupuncture and Moxibustion]	**Acupuncture:** Insert the needle perpendicularly 0.5~1.0 cun deep. **Moxibustion:** apply 3-5 moxa cones or needle-warming moxibustion or place a moxa stick above the point for 5-10 minutes.
[Indications]	Headache, heavy head, pain of the lower back, sacrum, hip, lateral thigh and knee.

GB-35 Yángjiāo — Xi-cleft point of the yang linking vessel

[Action]	Relaxes sinews and activates the collaterals and calms the spirit.
[Position]	On the lateral aspect of the lower limbs, 7 cun proximal to the tip of the external malleolus, on the posterior border of the fibula.
[Acupuncture and Moxibustion]	**Acupuncture:** Insert the needle perpendicularly 1.0~1.5 cun deep. **Moxibustion:** apply 3-5 moxa cones or needle-warming moxibustion or place a moxa stick above the point for 5-10 minutes.
[Indications]	Pain of the knee, atrophy or paralysis of the lower limbs, psychosis and sore throat.

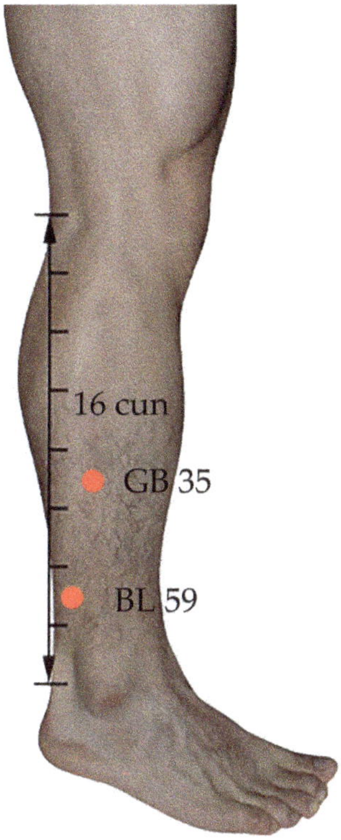

16 cun
GB 35
BL 59

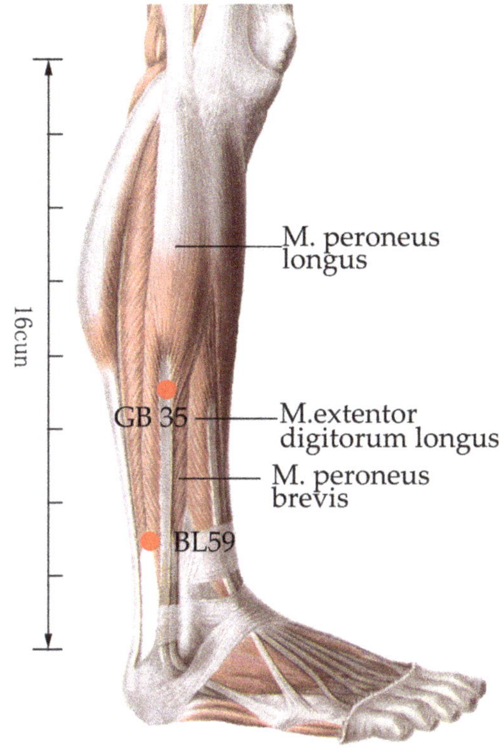

16cun
M. peroneus longus
GB 35
M.extentor digitorum longus
M. peroneus brevis
BL59

KI-8 Jiāoxìn — Xi-cleft point of the yin motility vessel

[Action]	Tonifies kidney and regulates menstruation, clears heat and induces diuresis.
[Position]	On the medial aspect of the lower leg, 2 cun superior to the tip of the medial ankle, in the depression posterior to the medial border of the tibia.
[Acupuncture and Moxibustion]	**Acupuncture:** Insert the needle perpendicularly 0.8~1.0 cun deep. **Moxibustion:** apply 3-5 moxa cones or needle-warming moxibustion or place a moxa stick above the point for 10-15 minutes.
[Indications]	Irregular menstruation, difficulty in stool, red-white dysentery, pain of the medial aspect of the lower extremity.

KI-9 Zhùbīn — Xi-cleft point of the yin linking vessel

[Action]	Tonifies and regulates liver and kidney, clears heart and transforms phlegm.
[Position]	On the medial side of the lower leg, 5 cun superior to KI 3 (Tàixī), between the belly of m. gastrocnemius and Achilles tendon
[Acupuncture and Moxibustion]	**Acupuncture:** Insert the needle perpendicularly 0.5~0.8 cun deep. **Moxibustion:** apply 3-5 moxa cones or needle-warming moxibustion or place a moxa stick above the point for 5-10 minutes.
[Indications]	Weakness and softness of the feet, pain on the medial aspect of the lower limbs.

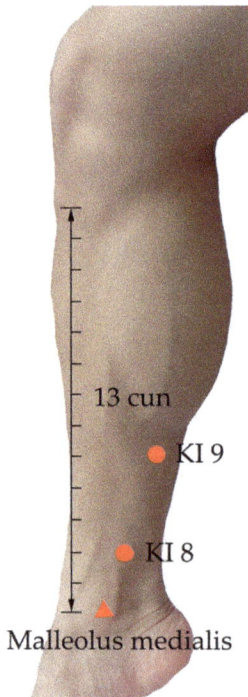

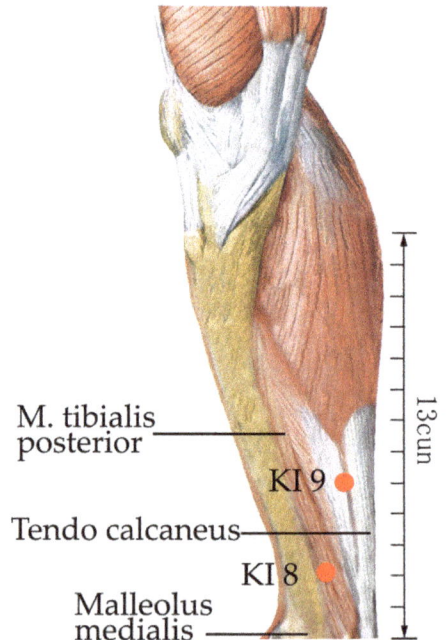

CHAPTER 10

Lower he-sea Points

ST-36 — Zúsānlǐ Lower he-sea point of ST

[Action]	Invigorates the spleen and harmonizes the stomach, prevents disease and benefits macrobiosis, dredges the channel and actives the collaterals, rises and falls Qi.
[Position]	On the anterior and lateral aspect of the lower leg, 3 cun distal to ST 35 (Dúbí), one finger width lateral from the anterior ridge of the tibia.
[Acupuncture and Moxibustion]	**Acupuncture:** Insert the needle perpendicularly 0.5~1.5 cun deep: **Moxibustion:** Apply 5-10 moxa cones or place a moxa stick above the point for 10~20 minutes.
[Indications]	Disorders of the stomach and intestines, disorders of the heart, wheezing with phlegm, carbuncle weakness, pain of the knee and shin pain, paralysis of the lower limbs, vertigo and disease of the eye.

ST-37 Shàngjùxū — Lower he-sea point of LI

[Action]	Regulates the spleen and stomach, dredges the channel and activates the collateral.
[Position]	On the anterior and lateral side of the leg, 6 cun distal to ST 35 (Dúbí), one finger width lateral from the anterior ridge of the tibia.
[Acupuncture and Moxibustion]	**Acupuncture:** Insert the needle perpendicularly1.0~2.0 cun deep: **Moxibustion:** Apply 5-9 moxa cones or needle-warming or place a moxa stick above the point for 10~20 minutes.
[Indications]	Diarrhea, constipation, borborygmus, abdominal distention and acute appendicitis.

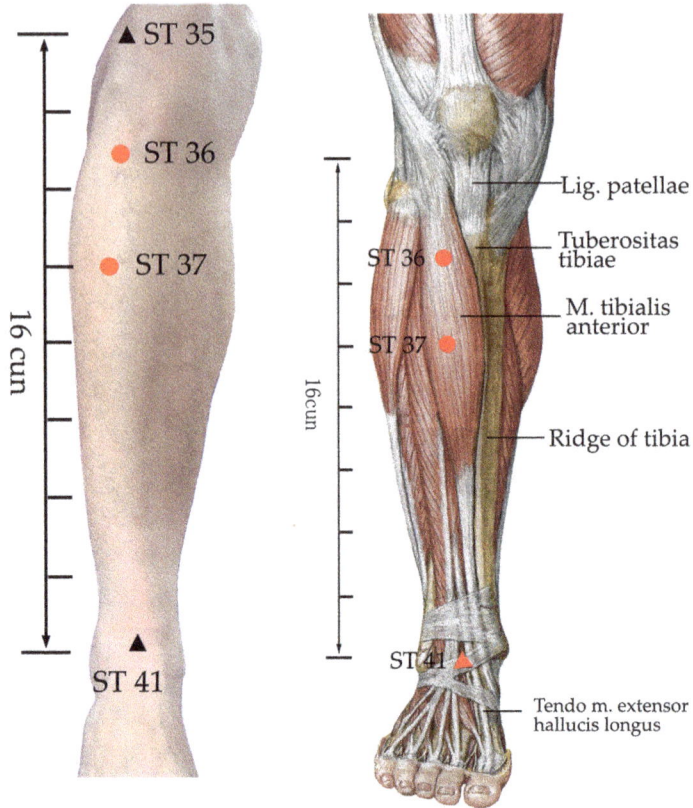

Labels on diagram:
- ▲ ST 35
- ST 36
- ST 37
- 16 cun
- ▲ ST 41
- Lig. patellae
- Tuberositas tibiae
- M. tibialis anterior
- ST 36
- 16cun
- ST 37
- Ridge of tibia
- ST 41
- Tendo m. extensor hallucis longus

ST-39 Xiàjùxū — Lower he-sea point of SI

[Action]	Regulates the spleen and stomach, dredges the channel and activates the collateral.
[Position]	On anterior and lateral side of the leg, 9 cun distal to ST 35 (Dúbí), one finger lateral to the anterior ridge of the tibia.
[Acupuncture and Moxibustion]	**Acupuncture:** Insert the needle perpendicularly 1.0~2.0 cun deep. **Moxibustion:** Apply 5-9 moxa cones or place a moxa stick above the point for 10~20 minutes.
[Indications]	Abdominal pain and borborygmus, diarrhoea, powerless and aches of the legs and knees.

GB-34 Yánglíngquán — Lower he-sea point of GB: He-sea point of GB: Influential point of the sinews

[Action]	Clears heat and pacifies wind, relieves swelling and alleviates pain.
[Position]	On the lateral aspect of the lower leg, in the depression anterior and inferior to the head of the fibula.
[Acupuncture and Moxibustion]	**Acupuncture:** Insert the needle perpendicularly towards SP9 (Yīnlíngquán) 1.0~3.0 cun deep **Moxibustion:** Apply 3-5moxa cones or place a moxa stick above the point for 5~10 minutes.
[Indications]	Headache, tinnitus, deafness, eye pain, swollen cheeks, pain of the chest and hypochondrium, swelling and pain of the breast, asthma, cough, chest distention, vomiting, jaundice, swelling and pain of the knee, weakness and numbness of the lower extremities, spasm, softness, contraction and tightness of the sinews, beriberi and hemiplegia.

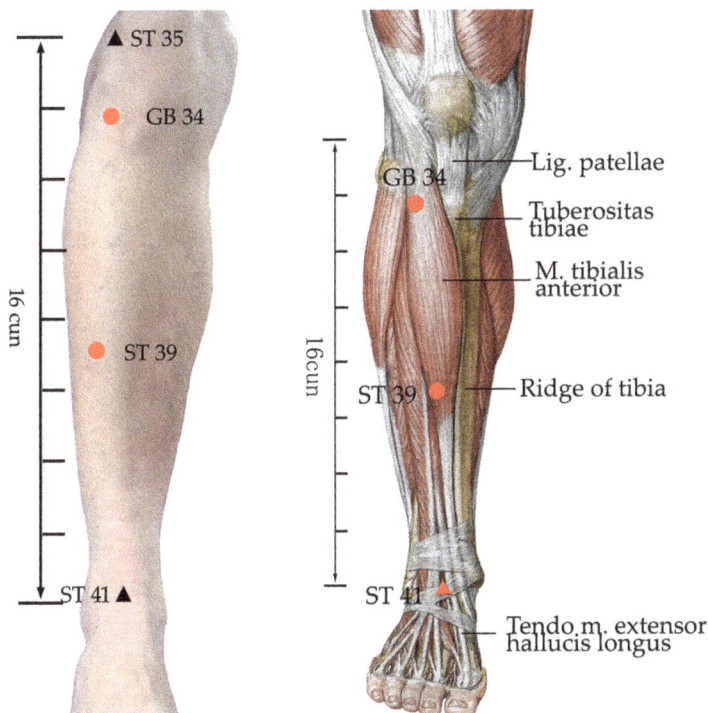

BL-40 Wěizhōng — He-sea point of BL: lower he-sea point of BL

[Action]	Clears summer heat, cools blood and detoxify, revives consciousness and calms heart, relaxes sinew and activates collaterals.
[Position]	At the midpoint of the transverse crease of the popliteal fossa, between the tendon of m. biceps femoris and m. semitendinous.
[Acupuncture and Moxibustion]	**Acupuncture:** Insert the needle perpendicularly 0.5~1.0 cun deep: Or prick with a three-edged needle to bleed. **Moxibustion:** Apply 5-7 moxa cones or place a moxa stick above the point for 10~20 minutes.
[Indications]	Lumbar pain, joint pain due to stagnation of damp-cold, weakness of the lower limbs, hemiplegia, beriberi, erysipelas, boils, furuncle, bruises and spontaneous bleeding under the skin, abdominal pain, vomiting and diarrhea.

BL-39 Wěiyáng — Lower he-sea point of TE

[Action]	Regulates sanjiao, relaxes sinews and dredges the collateral.
[Position]	At the lateral end of the popliteal transverse crease, on the medial side of the tendon of m. biceps femoris.
[Acupuncture and Moxibustion]	**Acupuncture:** Insert the needle perpendicularly 0.5~1.0 cun deep: **Moxibustion:** Apply 3-5 moxa cones or place a moxa stick above the point for 10~20 minutes.
[Indications]	Dribbling of urine, enuresis, urinary retention, edema and constipation, dysentery, chancre in children.

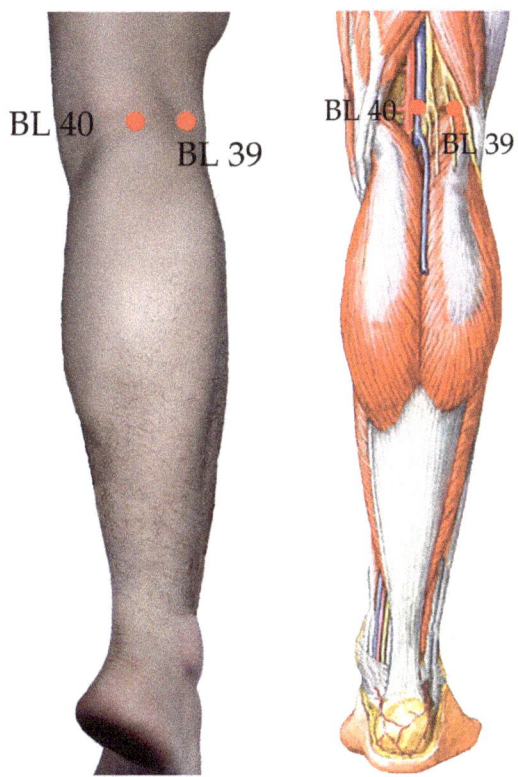

BL 40
BL 39
BL 40
BL 39

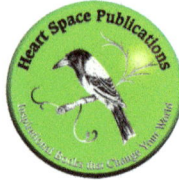

If you derived benefit from this manual,
please see the other three in the series of

Quick Reference Handbooks of Chinese Medicine

Acupuncture – of Acupoint Combinations Quick Lookups

Illustrations Of Special Effective Acupoints for common
Diseases

Human Body Reflex Zone Quick Lookup, Bilingual
anatomical illustration of reflex zones (English
edition)

Quick Investigation On Acupunture Points – Selection of
Professor Yang Jiasan

Go to www.heartspacepublications.com

www.ingramcontent.com/pod-product-compliance
Lightning Source LLC
Chambersburg PA
CBHW052012030426
42334CB00029BA/3191